# MCQs and
# Short Answer Questions
# for MRCOG

# MCQs and Short Answer Questions for MRCOG

An aid to revision and self-assessment

**Edited by**

**David M. Luesley** MA MD FRCOG
Lawson Tait Professor of Gynaecological Oncology, Department of Reproductive and Child Health, University of Birmingham, Birmingham; and Honorary Consultant Gynaecological Oncologist, Birmingham Women's Healthcare NHS Trust, Birmingham

*and*

**Philip N. Baker** DM BMedSci BM FRCOG
Professor of Maternal and Fetal Health, and Director of the Maternal and Fetal Health Research Centre, St Mary's Hospital, University of Manchester

*With additional contributions from*

**Jeremy C. Brockelsby** BSc MB BS PhD MRCOG
Clinical Lecturer in Obstetrics and Gynaecology, Maternal and Fetal Health Research Centre, St Mary's Hospital, University of Manchester

ARNOLD

A member of the Hodder Headline Group
LONDON

First published in Great Britain in 2004 by
Arnold, a member of the Hodder Headline Group,
338 Euston Road, London NW1 3BH

**http://www.arnoldpublishers.com**

Distributed in the United States of America by
Oxford University Press Inc.,
198 Madison Avenue, New York, NY10016
Oxford is a registered trademark of Oxford University Press

Whilst the advice and information in this book are believed to be true and
accurate at the date of going to press, neither the author[s] nor the publisher
can accept any legal responsibility or liability for any errors or omissions
that may be made. In particular (but without limiting the generality of the
preceding disclaimer) every effort has been made to check drug dosages;
however, it is still possible that errors have been missed. Furthermore,
dosage schedules are constantly being revised and new side-effects
recognized. For these reasons the reader is strongly urged to consult the
drug companies' printed instructions before administering any of the drugs
recommended in this book.

*British Library Cataloguing in Publication Data*
A catalogue record for this book is available from the British Library

*Library of Congress Cataloging-in-Publication Data*
A catalog record for this book is available from the Library of Congress

ISBN 0 340 80874 8
ISBN 0 340 88251 4 (International Students' Edition, restricted territorial availability)

1 2 3 4 5 6 7 8 9 10

| | |
|---|---|
| Commissioning Editor: | Joanna Koster |
| Development Editor: | Sarah Burrows |
| Project Editor: | Wendy Rooke |
| Production Controller: | Lindsay Smith |
| Cover Design: | Stuart Larking |
| Indexer: | Indexing Specialists (UK) Ltd |

618·0076 L

TO 6809

Typeset in 9 on 12pt Rotis Serif by Phoenix Photosetting, Chatham, Kent
Printed and bound in India

What do you think about this book? Or any other Arnold title?
Please send your comments to **feedback.arnold@hodder.co.uk**

# Contents

# Acknowledgements

The editors are grateful to the authors and section editors of the companion volume *Obstetrics and Gynaecology: An evidence-based text for MRCOG* for their help in compiling these true/false and short answer questions. The help of Drs Mires and Rabbani in ensuring the accuracy of the questions is also acknowledged.

Section Editors:
Linda Cardozo
James Drife
Lucy Kean
Mark D. Kilby
Henry C. Kitchener
William L. Ledger

Contributors:
James Balmforth, Margaret E. Cruickshank, Andrew Currie, Ian J. Etherington, Diana Fothergill, Harold Gee, Joanna C. Gillham, Barry W. Hancock, Richard Hayman, Susan J. Houghton, Tracey A. Johnston, Justin C. Konje, Sailesh Kumar, Hany A.M.A. Lashen, Murray Luckas, Melanie C. Mann, Pierre L. Martin-Hirsch, Alec McEwan, Enda McVeigh, Catherine Minto, Michele P. Mohajer, Catherine Nelson-Piercy, David Nunns, Michael E.L. Paterson, Charles Redman, Karina Reynolds, Dudley Robinson, Jane Rufford, Andrew Shennan, David Somerset, John Tidy, Peter J. Thompson

# Preface

This book of 'true/false' and 'short answer' questions is a companion text to *Obstetrics and Gynaecology: An evidence-based text for MRCOG*. When we compiled the MRCOG textbook, our aim was to move away from traditional or 'enteric-based' practice and attempt to detail the available evidence upon which our practice of obstetrics and gynaecology is based. The textbook template is linked to the MRCOG syllabus, in order to help trainees to understand the core knowledge of the specialty. The purpose of this companion volume is to assist the acquisition of 'evidence-based' core knowledge; this should be particularly valuable for candidates taking the membership examination.

Ideally, we suggest that readers work through each set of questions with pen and paper. We think that maximum benefit would be achieved if readers commit themselves on paper to the questions raised before referring to the subsequent answers. At the end of each question/group of questions, readers are referred to the appropriate chapter in the evidence-based textbook.

David M. Luesley and Philip N. Baker

# Glossary

| | |
|---|---|
| ABC | Airways, breathing and circulation |
| AC | Abdominal circumference |
| ACE | Angiotensin-converting enzyme |
| aCL | Anticardiolipin antibody |
| aFP | Alpha-fetoprotein |
| AIDS | Acquired immunodeficiency syndrome |
| AIMS | Association for Improvements in Maternity Services |
| AMH | Anti-Müllerian hormone |
| aPL | Antiphospholipid |
| APS | Antiphospholipid syndrome |
| AVM | Arteriovenous malformation |
| AZT | Zidovudine |
| bpm | Beats per minute |
| BPP | Biophysical profile |
| CEA | Carcinoembryonic antigen |
| CEMD | Confidential Enquiries into Maternal Deaths |
| CESDI | Confidential Enquiry into Stillbirths and Deaths in Infancy |
| CF | Cystic fibrosis |
| CI | Confidence interval |
| CIN | Cervical intraepithelial neoplasia |
| CMV | Cytomegalovirus |
| COCP | Combined oral contraceptive pill |
| COX-2 | Cyclo-oxygenase-2 |
| CPD | Cephalo-pelvic disproportion |
| CPS | Crown Prosecution Service |
| CRP | C-reactive protein |
| CT | Computed tomography |
| CTG | Cardiotocography |
| DDAVP | Desmopressin |
| DHEA | Dehydroepiandrosterone |
| DHEAS | Dehydroepiandrosterone sulphate |
| DVT | Deep vein thrombosis |
| EBV | Epstein–Barr virus |
| ECG | Electrocardiogram |
| ECV | External cephalic version |
| EFW | Estimated fetal weight |
| ER | [O]estrogen receptor |

| | |
|---|---|
| ESR | Erythrocyte sedimentation rate |
| FAS | Fetal alcohol syndrome |
| FSH | Follicle-stimulating hormone |
| GABA-A | Gamma-aminobutyric acid type A |
| GBS | Group B *Streptococcus* |
| GIFT | Gamete intrafallopian transfer |
| GnRH | Gonadotrophin releasing hormone |
| GUM | Genitourinary medicine |
| hCG | Human chorionic gonadotrophin |
| HDL | High-density lipoprotein |
| HELLP [syndrome] | Haemolysis, increased liver enzymes and low platelets |
| HFEA | Human Fertilisation and Embryology Authority |
| HIE | Hypoxic–ischaemic encephalopathy |
| HIV | Human immunodeficiency virus |
| HPV | Human papillomavirus |
| HRT | Hormone replacement therapy |
| HSG | Hysterosalpingogram |
| HSV | Herpes simplex virus |
| HWY | Hundred woman-years |
| IUCD | Intrauterine contraceptive device |
| IUGR | Intrauterine growth restriction |
| IVF | In-vitro fertilization |
| IVU | Intravenous urogram |
| IQ | Intelligence quotient |
| La | Lupus anticoagulant [antibodies] |
| LDL | Low-density lipoprotein |
| LFT | Liver function test |
| LH | Luteinizing hormone |
| LHRH | Luteinizing hormone releasing hormone |
| LLETZ | Large loop excision of the transformation zone |
| MCH | Mean corpuscular haemoglobin |
| MCHC | Mean cell haemoglobin concentration |
| MCV | Mean corpuscular volume |
| MIS | Müllerian inhibiting substance |
| MRI | Magnetic resonance imaging |
| MS | Multiple sclerosis |
| MSaFP | Maternal serum alpha-fetoprotein |
| MSU | Midstream urine |
| NAS | Neonatal abstinence syndrome |
| NCT | National Childbirth Trust |
| NHS | National Health Service |
| NICE | National Institute for Clinical Excellence |
| NSAID | Non-steroidal anti-inflammatory drug |
| NT | Nuchal translucency |

| | |
|---|---|
| NTD | Neural tube defect |
| OHSS | Ovarian hyperstimulation syndrome |
| OR | Odds ratio |
| PCOS | Polycystic ovarian syndrome |
| PCR | Polymerase chain reaction |
| PEP | Polymorphic eruption of pregnancy |
| PI | Pulsatility index |
| PID | Pelvic inflammatory disease |
| PMS | Premenstrual syndrome |
| POPQ | Pelvic Organ Prolapse Quantification [scoring system] |
| PR | Progesterone receptor |
| PPROM | Preterm pre-labour rupture of membranes |
| PROM | Pre-labour rupture of membranes |
| PTU | Propylthiouracil |
| RCOG | Royal College of Obstetricians and Gynaecologists |
| RCT | Randomized, controlled trial |
| Rh | Rhesus |
| SD | Standard deviation |
| SERM | Selective [o]estrogen receptor modulator |
| SHBG | Sex hormone-binding globulin |
| SLE | Systemic lupus erythematosus |
| STD | Sexually transmitted disease |
| STI | Sexually transmitted infection |
| T3 | Triiodothyronine |
| T4 | Thyroxine |
| TB | Tuberculosis |
| TED | Thromboembolic deterrent [stocking] |
| TSH | Thyroid-stimulating hormone |
| TTTS | Twin–twin transfusion syndrome |
| TVT | Tension-free vaginal tape |
| TVUS | Transvaginal ultrasound |
| UTI | Urinary tract infection |
| VIN | Vulval intraepithelial neoplasia |
| VMA | Vanillylmandelic acid |
| V/Q | Ventilation/perfusion [scan] |
| VTE | Venous thromboembolism |
| WCC | White cell count |
| WHO | World Health Organization |

# Multiple Choice Questions

# OBSTETRICS

**1. In chronic hypertension in pregnancy:**
A. The perinatal risk is only increased in the presence of proteinuria.
B. The use of thiazide diuretics is associated with teratogenesis.
C. First trimester use of angiotensin-converting enzyme (ACE) inhibitors is an indication for a termination of pregnancy.
D. Methyldopa is free of side effects.
E. The relative risk of pre-eclampsia supervening is more than doubled.
*See Chapter 6.1, Chronic hypertension.*

**2. When treating moderate hypertension in pregnancy:**
A. The risk of pre-eclampsia is reduced.
B. The risk of severe hypertension is reduced.
C. There is an increase in birth weight.
D. Calcium channel blockers are contraindicated as they have tocolytic effects.
E. Treatment should be discontinued 24 hours after delivery.
*See Chapter 6.1, Chronic hypertension.*

**3. With regard to chronic hypertension:**
A. It affects 0.1 per cent of pregnant women.
B. ACE inhibitors are associated with fetal renal failure.
C. Labetolol is associated with intrauterine growth restriction (IUGR).
D. Fifty per cent of affected women will develop superimposed pre-eclampsia.
E. The second most common complication is placental abruption.
*See Chapter 6.1, Chronic hypertension.*

**4. With regard to the management of diabetes mellitus in pregnancy:**
A. Frequent umbilical Doppler velocimetry will reduce the perinatal mortality rate.
B. A rise in insulin requirements at term is a poor prognostic sign.
C. Caesarean section is indicated if the estimated fetal weight is >3.5 kg.
D. Polyhydramnios can be prevented by insulin therapy.
*See Chapter 6.2, Diabetes mellitus.*

### 5.  With regard to diabetes mellitus:

A. It complicates 1–2 per cent of pregnancies in the UK.

B. The complication of diabetic ketoacidosis is associated with a 50 per cent fetal mortality rate.

C. A maternal four-dose insulin regimen gives better maternal and fetal outcomes than a two-dose regimen.

D. In poorly controlled women the risk of fetal polyhydramnios is 25–30 per cent.

E. The congenital malformation rate is five to ten times that of non-diabetic pregnancies.

  *See Chapter 6.2, Diabetes mellitus.*

### 6.  The infant of a diabetic mother is at increased risk of:

A. Polycythaemia.

B. Hypermagnesaemia.

C. Traumatic delivery.

D. Neonatal jaundice.

E. Hypoglycaemia.

  *See Chapter 6.2, Diabetes mellitus.*

### 7.  The following conditions are contraindications to pregnancy:

A. Wolf–Parkinson–White syndrome.

B. Eisenmenger's syndrome.

C. Mild mitral stenosis.

D. Primary pulmonary hypertension.

E. Marfan's syndrome with a dilated aortic root.

  *See Chapter 6.3, Cardiac disease.*

### 8.  With regard to peripartum cardiomyopathy:

A. It usually occurs in the last month of pregnancy.

B. Risk factors include multiple pregnancy, hypertension and nulliparity.

C. Cardiac transplantation is inappropriate.

D. Anticoagulation is required.

E. Cerebral embolization is a major cause of morbidity.

  *See Chapter 6.3, Cardiac disease.*

### 9.  Pregnancy is associated with:

A. Increased thyroid-binding globulin.

B. Increased free thyroxine (T4).

C. Increased free triiodothyronine (T3).

D. Decreased maternal iodide levels.

E. Increased total T4.

  *See Chapter 6.4, Thyroid disease.*

**10.  Propylthiouracil (PTU) therapy for a pregnant woman with Graves' disease:**

A. Reduces the titre of thyroid-stimulating hormone (TSH) receptor antibodies.

B. Inhibits the peripheral conversion of T3 to T4.

C. Is associated with teratogenesis.

D. Can cause agranulocytosis.

   *See Chapter 6.4, Thyroid disease.*

**11.  Untreated hypothyroidism in pregnancy is associated with:**

A. Weight gain, hyperactivity, tachycardia.

B. Increased rate of miscarriage, pre-eclampsia and low-birth-weight babies.

C. An increased risk of congenital anomalies.

D. Reduced intelligence quotient (IQ) in infants.

E. Delayed infant neurodevelopment.

   *See Chapter 6.4, Thyroid disease.*

**12.  With regard to venous thromboembolism in pregnancy:**

A. Deep venous thromboses (DVTs) usually occur in the right leg.

B. Duplex ultrasound is sensitive for deep venous thromboses in the proximal leg.

C. A chest X-ray should routinely be performed when investigating chest pain in the second and third trimester.

D. Intravenous heparin is the first choice of treatment in the acute presentation of a deep venous thrombosis.

E. Thrombolysis is contraindicated in pregnancy.

   *See Chapter 6.5, Haematological conditions.*

**13.  With regard to haemophilia A and B:**

A. They are autosomal recessive diseases.

B. Haemophilia B results from factor IX deficiency.

C. Female carriers usually have normal factor VIII levels in haemophilia.

D. Caesarean section is the usual mode of delivery in haemophilia pregnancies.

E. Desmopressin (DDAVP) is used to increase factor IX levels.

   *See Chapter 6.5, Haematological conditions.*

**14.  In maternal sickle cell disease:**

A. The spontaneous abortion rate is increased.

B. The incidence of pre-eclampsia is increased.

C. The incidence of spontaneous delivery preterm is increased.

D. The incidence of small-for-dates fetuses is unchanged.

E. Sickle cell disease cannot be diagnosed in the fetus.

   *See Chapter 6.5, Haematological conditions.*

**15. The following are indicative of underlying pre-existing renal disease:**
A. Bilateral renal pelvi-calyceal dilatation on ultrasound.
B. Bilateral small kidneys on ultrasound.
C. Trace proteinuria and 1+ haematuria at booking at 10 weeks.
D. A serum creatinine of 99 μmol/L at 16 weeks in a woman weighing 59 kg.
E. A 24-hour urinary protein loss of 3.5 g at 12 weeks.
*See Chapter 6.6, Renal disease.*

**16. Concerning bacteriuria in pregnancy:**
A. Asymptomatic bacteriuria complicates about 1 per cent of pregnancies.
B. Bacteriuria is considered significant if there are more than 10 000 organisms per mL of urine.
C. A 7-day course of antibiotics is recommended for asymptomatic bacteriuria.
D. A 7-day course of antibiotics is recommended for pyelonephritis.
E. Nitrofurantoin therapy should be avoided in the first trimester.
*See Chapter 6.6, Renal disease (and Chapter 6.2, Diabetes mellitus).*

**17. Proteinuria in pregnancy may be due to:**
A. The presence of systemic lupus erythematosus (SLE).
B. Diabetes mellitus.
C. Chronic glomerulonephritis.
D. Placental abruption without pre-eclampsia.
E. Essential benign hypertension.
*See Chapter 6.6, Renal disease (and Chapter 6.2, Diabetes mellitus).*

**18. The following drugs are appropriate for a woman with SLE who is 35 weeks pregnant:**
A. Diclofenac.
B. Prednisolone.
C. Hydroxychloroquine.
D. Sulfasalazine.
E. Methotrexate.
*See Chapter 6.7, Autoimmune conditions.*

**19. A woman with a previous stillbirth and a postpartum DVT is found to have lupus anticoagulant and medium-titre immunoglobulin M (IgM) anticardiolipin antibodies (aCL) on two occasions. In a subsequent pregnancy:**
A. She has an increased risk of miscarriage.
B. Low-dose aspirin should be discontinued at 34 weeks.
C. Warfarin should be discontinued.
D. She does not require postpartum heparin if she has a vaginal delivery.
E. She requires antibiotic prophylaxis to cover delivery.
*See Chapter 6.7, Autoimmune conditions.*

### 20.  With regard to antiphospholipid syndrome (APS):

A. It may be diagnosed if aCL or lupus anticoagulant (La) antibodies are detected in a woman who has suffered a miscarriage at less than 10 weeks.
B. It increases the risk of placental abruption.
C. Previous pregnancy outcome is the best predictor of present pregnancy outcome.
D. Fetal death is typically preceded by IUGR and oligohydramnios.
E. High-dose steroid therapy is a recommended treatment.

*See Chapter 6.7, Autoimmune conditions.*

### 21.  With regard to SLE:

A. There is an increased likelihood of an exacerbation during pregnancy.
B. There is an increased prevalence in Caucasian women.
C. The C-reactive protein (CRP) level is raised.
D. Anti-double-stranded DNA is the most common autoantibody.
E. Anti-Ro antibodies are present in 30 per cent of women with SLE.

*See Chapter 6.7, Autoimmune conditions.*

### 22.  In a women with obstetric cholestasis:

A. The risk of stillbirth increases with gestation.
B. The presence of steatorrhoea increases the risk of postpartum haemorrhage.
C. The pruritus may recur with use of the combined oral contraceptive pill (COCP).
D. Recurrence in subsequent pregnancies is unlikely.
E. The treatment of choice is cholestyramine.

*See Chapter 6.8, Liver and gastrointestinal disease.*

### 23.  Intrahepatic cholestasis in pregnancy is associated with:

A. Elevation of total bile salts in the blood.
B. A positive direct Coombs' test in the neonate.
C. Elevated serum acid phosphatase activity.
D. Preterm labour.
E. Marked geographical variations.

*See Chapter 6.8, Liver and gastrointestinal disease.*

### 24.  Recognized causes of vomiting in the second trimester of pregnancy include:

A. Ectopic pregnancy.
B. Herpes gestationis.
C. Ulcerative colitis.
D. Acute pyelonephritis.
E. Appendicitis.

*See Chapter 6.8, Liver and gastrointestinal disease.*

## 25. Regarding respiratory disease in pregnancy:

A. Theophyllines are contraindicated in pregnancy.

B. Pregnancy does not cause a net deterioration of cystic fibrosis.

C. Congenital tuberculosis occurs in 25 per cent of cases of maternal tuberculosis (TB).

D. Aciclovir should be given within 24 hours of a chickenpox rash developing.

E. Women being treated for TB should be advised not to breastfeed.

*See Chapter 6.9, Respiratory conditions.*

## 26. With regard to tuberculosis:

A. It is caused by the organism *Mycobacterium tuberculosis*.

B. Delayed treatment in pregnancy is associated with IUGR.

C. Delayed treatment in pregnancy is associated with prematurity.

D. Vertical transmission to the fetus is common.

E. Separation of the infant from the mother is usually necessary to prevent lateral transmission.

F. The drugs isoniazid, ethambutol and streptomycin are safe in pregnancy.

*See Chapter 6.9, Respiratory conditions.*

## 27. A 28-year-old woman has cystic fibrosis (CF) and her partner is negative for the common ΔF 508 mutation. With regard to her pregnancy:

A. The risk of their offspring being affected with CF is 1:5000.

B. Colonization with *Burkholderia cepacia* is a predictor of maternal pregnancy outcome.

C. An oral glucose tolerance test should be arranged at 26 weeks.

D. There is, on average, a 30 per cent loss of lung function with pregnancy.

E. She has only a 40 per cent chance of being alive 10 years after giving birth.

*See Chapter 6.9, Respiratory conditions.*

## 28. Regarding neurological disease in pregnancy:

A. The overall progression of multiple sclerosis (MS) is accelerated by pregnancy.

B. Women using benzodiazepines in pregnancy should receive vitamin K supplements.

C. Neonatal myasthenia occurs in no more than 50 per cent of babies born to women with myasthenia gravis.

D. The pregnancy-associated increase in stroke risk is mostly confined to the puerperium.

E. Arteriovenous malformations are a more common cause of intracerebral haemorrhage than aneurysms.

*See Chapter 6.10, Neuromuscular conditions.*

## 29. Regarding MS:

A. Pregnancy affects the long-term prognosis of the disease.

B. Epidural analgesia will precipitate a relapse.

C. Attacks are more likely to occur in pregnancy.

D. Urinary urgency may be treated with tricyclic antidepressants.

E. The infant has a 10 per cent risk of developing MS later in life.

*See Chapter 6.10, Neuromuscular conditions.*

**30. In relation to women who embark on pregnancy with a diagnosis of epilepsy:**

A. Carbamazepine is associated with fetal cardiac defects.

B. Following delivery, anti-epileptic drugs may need to be reduced.

C. Vitamin K should be commenced from 30 weeks' gestation.

D. Maternal death via drowning is a recognized association of epilepsy.

E. Intravenous magnesium sulphate is the best treatment of a status epilepticus during labour.

*See Chapter 6.10, Neuromuscular conditions.*

**31. Polymorphic eruption of pregnancy (PEP) is associated with:**

A. Increased rates of stillbirth.

B. Approximately 1:250 pregnancies.

C. A typical onset in the second trimester.

D. No fetal effects.

E. Recurrence in subsequent pregnancies.

*See Chapter 6.11, Dermatological conditions.*

**32. With regard to dermatological conditions in pregnancy:**

A. PEP is characterized by an abdominal rash with umbilical sparing.

B. Erythema nodosum may deteriorate or present in pregnancy.

C. Podophyllin does not cross the placenta in clinically significant amounts.

*See Chapter 6.11, Dermatological conditions.*

**33. Regarding substance misuse in pregnancy:**

A. Neonatal abstinence syndrome (NAS) does not occur with methadone use.

B. Cocaine acts via the central gamma-aminobutyric acid type A (GABA-A) receptor to cause hypertension.

C. A third of alcoholics produce offspring with the fetal alcohol syndrome (FAS).

D. A clear causal link exists between benzodiazepine exposure in the first trimester and cleft lip and palate.

E. Marijuana causes fetal microcephaly.

*See Chapter 6.12, Drug and alcohol misuse.*

**34. With regard to substance abuse:**

A. Cannabis smoking is associated with IUGR.

B. Cocaethylene is a potent vasoconstrictor derived from cocaine.

C. Alcohol has abortive properties.

D. Cocaine is associated with macrocephaly.

E. Benzodiazepines in the neonate cause respiratory depression, reduced tone and poor feeding.

*See Chapter 6.12, Drug and alcohol misuse.*

**35.  Regarding methadone use in pregnancy:**
A. Methadone has a shorter half-life than heroin.
B. Naloxone should not be given to opiate-dependent mothers or their offspring.
C. NAS presents within 24 hours of delivery.
D. Breastfeeding is contraindicated.

*See Chapter 6.12, Drug and alcohol misuse.*

**36.  Smoking in pregnancy is associated with increased risks of:**
A. Premature labour.
B. Long-term respiratory disease amongst infants.
C. Lowered IQs amongst offspring.

*See Chapter 6.13, Smoking.*

**37.  Smoking in pregnancy is associated with:**
A. An increase in the incidence of pre-eclampsia.
B. A reduction in cognitive function for the infant later in life.
C. A reduction in the infant birth weight.
D. An increase in postoperative chest infections.
E. An increase in the rate of placental abruption.

*See Chapter 6.13, Smoking.*

**38.  Pregnancy is associated with increases in:**
A. Total iron-binding capacity.
B. Iron absorption.
C. Haematocrit.
D. Mean cell haemoglobin concentration (MCHC).
E. Serum ferritin concentration.

*See Chapter 7.1, Anaemia.*

**39.  In pregnancy:**
A. A haemoglobin concentration of 11 g/dL is the lower limit of normal according to the World Health Organization (WHO).
B. A low serum iron with a low total iron-binding capacity suggests iron deficiency.
C. The overall total iron requirement is approximately 1000 mg.
D. Iron absorption from the jejunum is increased.
E. Iron should be advised for all pregnant women.

*See Chapter 7.1, Anaemia.*

**40.  With regard to acute appendicitis in pregnancy:**
A. It is more common than outside pregnancy.
B. It is associated with preterm rupture of membranes.
C. Caesarean section should not be performed at the same time as an appendicectomy.
D. Maternal mortality exceeds 5 per cent.

*See Chapter 7.2, Abdominal pain.*

**41. With regard to abdominal pain in the third trimester of pregnancy:**

A. An ultrasound scan can exclude a placental abruption.

B. Appendicitis is characterized by maximum tenderness over McBurney's point.

C. Round ligament pain is the most common cause.

D. Acute pyelonephritis is more likely on the left than on the right.

*See Chapter 7.2, Abdominal pain.*

**42. Regarding cancer arising during pregnancy:**

A. Chemotherapy must never be given during the first trimester.

B. The long-term survival after diagnosis of melanoma is adversely affected by pregnancy.

C. The maximum recommended radiation exposure during pregnancy is 5 Gray.

D. Treatment of cervical intraepithelial neoplasia (CIN) is usually delayed until after delivery.

E. Breast cancer is the most common cancer to be diagnosed during pregnancy.

*See Chapter 7.3, Malignancy.*

**43. With regard to cancer in pregnancy:**

A. Twenty-five per cent of cancers presenting in pregnancy are breast cancers.

B. Technetium bone scans are indicated.

C. Radical hysterectomy is mandatory for micro-invasive cervical cancer.

D. Cervical cancer is an indication for a classical caesarean section.

E. Hodgkin's lymphoma must be treated immediately upon diagnosis.

*See Chapter 7.3, Malignancy.*

**44. With regard to human immunodeficiency virus (HIV) in pregnancy:**

A. A positive HIV blood test in pregnancy is not reliable.

B. A low maternal CD4 count increases the mother-to-child transmission of HIV.

C. A high maternal HIV RNA load increases the mother-to-child transmission of HIV.

D. Use of antiretroviral agents is always commenced in the first trimester of pregnancy.

E. HIV infection increases the mother-to child transmission of the hepatitis C virus.

F. If there are ruptured membranes for 6 hours, there is no advantage to delivery by caesarean section.

*See Chapter 7.4, Infection.*

**45. With regard to viral infection in pregnancy:**

A. The majority of genital herpes is caused by type 2 herpes simplex virus (HSV).

B. Initial treatment for HSV in pregnancy should include a penicillin.

C. Shingles in pregnancy does not appear to cause fetal sequelae.

D. Cytomegalovirus (CMV) is associated with non-immune fetal hydrops.

*See Chapter 7.4, Infection.*

### 46. Chlamydial infection in pregnancy:
A. Has an incubation period of up to 21 days.
B. Is typically asymptomatic.
C. Can present with perihepatitis.
D. Should be treated with tetracycline.
E. Can cause postpartum endometritis.
   *See Chapter 7.4, Infection.*

### 47. Congenital infection with CMV:
A. Is associated with hepatosplenomegaly.
B. Is associated with intracerebral calcification.
C. Is a cause of microcephaly.
D. Will result in symptoms in 5–10 per cent of babies at birth.
E. Is a cause of polyhydramnios.
   *See Chapter 7.4, Infection.*

### 48. *Listeria monocytogenes*:
A. Is a Gram-negative anaerobe.
B. Is carried in the intestinal tract of 20 per cent of the population.
C. Is spread through droplets in the air.
D. Is a spore-forming bacterium.
E. Is associated with meconium staining of the liquor amnii in premature gestations.
   *See Chapter 7.4, Infection.*

### 49. Gestational diabetes diagnosed for the first time during pregnancy is characteristically associated with:
A. An increased risk of developing diabetes mellitus later in life.
B. A need for treatment with insulin in the majority of cases.
C. An increased incidence of fetal malformations, even when treated.
D. A decreased risk of pre-eclampsia.
E. An increased risk of fetal respiratory distress syndrome.
   *See Chapter 7.5, Gestational diabetes.*

### 50. Screening tests for diabetes in pregnancy include:
A. Performing glycosylated haemoglobin estimations on all women who have had a macrosomic baby (>4.5 kg).
B. Random blood sampling at 28–32 weeks.
C. A 50 g glucose load at booking.
D. A 50 g glucose load at 28 weeks if potential diabetic features pertain.
E. Glucose testing of the urine.
   *See Chapter 7.5, Gestational diabetes.*

**51.  The incidence of pre-eclampsia is:**

A. Increased in teenage pregnancies.

B. Increased in pregnancies complicated by hydrops fetalis.

C. Doubled by a family history in a first-degree relative.

D. Increased in women with gestational diabetes.

E. Approximately 20 per cent if there is notching on uterine artery Doppler waveform analysis at 20 weeks.

F. Reduced by prophylactic fish oil administration.

*See Chapter 7.6, Pre-eclampsia and non-proteinuric pregnancy-induced hypertension.*

**52.  With regard to eclampsia:**

A. Eighteen per cent of eclamptic seizures occur in the postnatal period.

B. Magnesium sulphate administration is associated with fetal hypercalcaemia.

C. Magnesium sulphate can only be given intravenously.

D. The commonest cause of maternal death is cerebral vascular accident.

E. It is a recognized cause of cortical blindness.

*See Chapter 7.6, Pre-eclampsia and non-proteinuric pregnancy-induced hypertension.*

**53.  In HELLP (haemolysis, increased liver enzymes and low platelets) syndrome:**

A. Most patients are in the immediate postpartum state.

B. Platelet count falls below $100 \times 10^9/L$.

C. The recurrence rate is 40–60 per cent if the index pregnancy diagnosis was after 32 weeks.

D. The lactate dehydrogenase concentration falls.

E. Profound vasodilatation occurs.

*See Chapter 7.6, Pre-eclampsia and non-proteinuric pregnancy-induced hypertension.*

**54.  Concerning the administration of drugs in pregnancy:**

A. Highly lipid-soluble drugs administered via the respiratory system reach higher concentrations in the plasma at a faster rate in pregnant than in non-pregnant women.

B. Anti-metabolites administered in pregnancy are associated with preterm labour.

C. Carbamazepine is the safest anticonvulsant agent in pregnancy.

D. When administered in the third trimester, beta-blockers may cause fetal hyperglycaemia.

E. When cholera vaccines are administered in the first trimester, termination of pregnancy should be offered.

F. Acetaminophen (paracetamol) is considered the analgesic of choice in pregnancy.

*See Chapter 8, Medication in pregnancy.*

**55.  The following are teratogenic consequences of drug administration in pregnancy:**

A. Tetracycline: yellowish coloration of the teeth.

B. Phenytoin: cleft lip and palate.

C. Sodium valproate: neural tube defects (NTDs).

D. Heparin: nasal hypoplasia.

E. Zidovudine (AZT): skull defects.

F. Penicillin: cardiac defects.

*See Chapter 8, Medication in pregnancy.*

**56. Concerning the use of antibiotics in pregnancy:**

A. Erythromycin does not cross the placenta.

B. Trimethoprim is associated with the neonatal grey baby syndrome.

C. Streptomycin is associated with sensorineural deafness.

D. Erythromycin is the drug of choice in patients with premature rupture of fetal membranes.

E. Cephalosporins are associated with neonatal jaundice.

*See Chapter 8, Medication in pregnancy.*

**57. The following drugs are correctly paired with the following complications:**

A. Carbimazole: fetal goitre.

B. Warfarin: fetal chondrodysplasia.

C. Labetalol: IUGR.

D. Sodium valproate: NTDs.

E. Lithium: cardiac malformations.

*See Chapter 8, Medication in pregnancy.*

**58. With regard to maternal mortalities:**

A. They include those deaths caused by ectopic pregnancies.

B. Forty per cent of the maternal deaths in the UK occur in social class 1.

C. Their incidence is higher in patients over the age of 40.

D. Epilepsy is the commonest cause of indirect maternal death.

E. In the UK, Asian women have a reduced likelihood of death in pregnancy in comparison to Caucasian women.

*See Chapter 9, Maternal mortality.*

**59. From data for the UK from the 2001 Confidential Enquiry into Stillbirths and Deaths in Infancy (CESDI):**

A. Congenital anomalies are responsible for 1 in 5 pregnancy losses.

B. Abruptio placentae is associated with 50 per cent of stillbirths.

C. Intrapartum asphyxia is responsible for 20 per cent of fetal deaths.

D. The largest percentage is 'unexplained'.

*See Chapter 11, Previous history of fetal loss.*

**60. With regard to APS:**

A. It may be associated with unexplained stillbirth.

B. A single positive aCL titre is diagnostic of this condition.

C. Association with pulmonary hypertension is of little consequence.

D. Aspirin alone is the pharmacotherapy of choice.

*See Chapter 11, Previous history of fetal loss.*

### 61.  In monochorionic pregnancies:

A. There are intraplacental vascular anastomoses.

B. Perinatal mortality is increased after 28 weeks.

C. A discordancy in first trimester nuchal translucency could denote different risks of aneuploidy.

D. There is a lower risk of twin–twin transfusion syndrome (TTTS) than in dichorionic twinning.

E. Twins are always monozygous.

*See Chapter 12, Multiple pregnancy.*

### 62.  In TTTS:

A. The smaller twin is the recipient.

B. The smaller twin has the greatest risk of cardiac compromise.

C. The larger twin is often 'stuck' to the uterine wall.

D. Serial amnioreduction improves perinatal survival.

E. Fetoscopic laser ablation of the placental vessels increases survival for both twins.

*See Chapter 12, Multiple pregnancy.*

### 63.  In ultrasound screening for chorionicity:

A. The sensitivity and specificity of defining chorionicity are improved after 16 weeks' gestation.

B. A 'twin peak' or 'lambda sign' is associated with dichorionicity.

C. A thick dividing amniotic membrane is present in monochorionicity.

D. Same fetal sex excludes dichorionicity.

E. A single placental mass is indicative of monochorionicity in the first trimester.

*See Chapter 12, Multiple pregnancy.*

### 64.  With regard to CMV:

A. It is an RNA virus.

B. It causes primary infection in 25–40 per cent of cases.

C. It may cause fetal IUGR.

D. Ganciclovir administered to the fetus has proven efficacy – demonstrated in randomized, controlled trials (RCTs).

E. It is associated with cerebral calcification.

*See Chapter 13, Fetal infections.*

### 65.  Human parvovirus B19:

A. Is a DNA virus.

B. Is transmitted as a respiratory infection of children.

C. Has an incubation period of up to 6 weeks.

D. Has predilection to fetal erythrocyte progenitor cells.

E. Crosses the placenta in <10 per cent of cases.

*See Chapter 13, Fetal infections.*

**66. With regard to antenatal cardiotocography (CTG):**

A. One acceleration of heart rate 15 beats per minute (bpm) above the baseline lasting 15 seconds is reassuring.

B. Vibroacoustic stimulation reduces the number of unreactive traces.

C. It is more predictive of fetal death than absent end-diastolic umbilical artery Doppler velocimetry.

D. It has a strong effect on improved perinatal mortality.

*See Chapter 14, Tests of fetal well-being.*

**67. The ultrasound biophysical profile (BPP):**

A. Has a low false-negative rate.

B. Has a predictive negative value of 35 per cent for perinatal mortality.

C. Includes liquor volume assessment as part of the test.

D. Has proven value in preventing perinatal mortality in RCTs.

*See Chapter 14, Tests of fetal well-being.*

**68. Ultrasound parameters indicative of fetal growth restriction include:**

A. Oligohydramnios.

B. A symphysis–fundal height <3rd centile.

C. An abdominal circumference (AC) <10th centile.

D. Aberrant middle cerebral artery to umbilical artery Doppler pulsatility index (PI) ratio.

E. A change in growth velocity ($\delta$AC <1 standard deviation (SD) in 14 days).

*See Chapter 15, Fetal growth restriction.*

**69. With regard to fetal growth restriction:**

A. The perinatal mortality is lower for gestational age than for appropriately grown babies.

B. There is a decreased risk of pulmonary haemorrhage in neonatal life.

C. It may be associated with elevated maternal serum alpha-fetoprotein (aFP) and beta-human chorionic gonadotrophin ($\beta$hCG).

D. It is more sensitively detected using customized growth charts.

*See Chapter 15, Fetal growth restriction.*

**70. Oligohydramnios:**

A. Is commonly associated with amniorrhexis.

B. Is associated at 16 weeks with a >90 per cent risk of pulmonary hypoplasia.

C. May cause postural anomalies in the fetus.

D. Is commonly found in diabetic pregnancies.

*See Chapter 16, Abberant liquor volume.*

**71. With regard to polyhydramnios:**

A. Increased amniotic fluid index has a detrimental effect on uterine blood flow.

B. It may be associated with fetal oesophageal atresia.

C. It is commonly associated with the 'donor' twin in TTTS.

D. It may be safely managed with indomethacin in the third trimester.

E. It is diagnosed in 3 per cent of all pregnancies.

*See Chapter 16, Abberant liquor volume.*

**72. Fetal hydrops is commonly caused by:**

A. Anti-Duffy antibodies.

B. Maternal human parvovirus B19 infection.

C. Fetal tachydysrhythmias.

D. Fetal akinesia syndromes.

*See Chapter 17, Fetal hydrops.*

**73. Fetal hydrops can be caused by:**

A. Increased fetal hydrostatic pressure.

B. Reduced oncotic pressure.

C. Fetal tumours.

D. Fetal polycythaemia.

*See Chapter 17, Fetal hydrops.*

**74. For term breech presentations:**

A. The incidence is 3–4 per cent.

B. Planned caesarean delivery reduces perinatal morbidity by 75 per cent.

C. Caesarean section has been shown to reduce perinatal morbidity in those presenting in labour.

D. All women should be offered external cephalic version (ECV).

*See Chapter 18, Malpresentation.*

**75. With regard to ECV for term breech presentation:**

A. Fetal heart activity should be documented.

B. Tocolysis is always required.

C. It is less likely to be successful in a multiparous woman.

D. It reduces the need for caesarean section.

E. Anti-D should be administered to Rhesus-negative women.

*See Chapter 18, Malpresentation.*

### 76. Prolonged pregnancy:

A. Occurs in between 8 and 14 per cent of pregnancies.
B. Is associated with an increased risk of stillbirth after 43 weeks.
C. Is associated with an increase risk of maternal haemorrhage.
D. Should be managed by induction of labour at 41+ weeks.
E. Incidence is reduced with early ultrasound dating.

*See Chapter 19, Prolonged pregnancy.*

### 77. The following interventions are supported by high-grade evidence to reduce surgical intervention in low-risk labour:

A. Preparation and support of the woman in labour.
B. Routine amniotomy.
C. Epidural analgesia.
D. Presence of 'Doula' support.
E. Continuous electronic fetal heart rate monitoring.

*See Chapter 20, Routine intrapartum care: an overview.*

### 78. Cervicography gives:

A. Reliable information in the latent phase.
B. Reliable information in the active phase.
C. Prospective identification of aberrant progress.
D. Diagnosis of underlying pathology when there is poor progress.
E. Good predictive value for operative delivery (2-hour action line).

*See Chapter 20, Routine intrapartum care: an overview.*

### 79. The following are of proven benefit with regard to preterm labour:

A. Oral metronidazole in women at high risk of preterm labour who are positive for bacterial vaginosis.
B. Treatment of asymptomatic bacteriuria with antibiotics.
C. Hospitalization for bed rest for women at high risk.
D. Antibiotics for women presenting with threatened preterm labour with intact membranes.
E. Oral tocolysis in women at high risk of preterm labour.
F. Antenatal treatment of group B *Streptococcus* (GBS).

*See Chapter 21, Preterm labour.*

### 80. With regard to preterm labour:

A. The rate of severe handicap for infants delivered at 24–26 weeks is 25 per cent.
B. The risk of preterm labour is inversely proportional to cervical length.
C. Digital cervical length assessment is as clinically useful as ultrasound assessment.
D. Home uterine activity monitoring is ineffective in reducing the risk of preterm labour.
E. Tocolysis for threatened preterm labour reduces the risk of delivery within 48 hours.

*See Chapter 21, Preterm labour.*

## 81. With regard to pre-labour rupture of membranes (PROM) at term:

A. Ninety per cent of women will labour within 24 hours.

B. Ultrasound is not a useful primary test in establishing the diagnosis.

C. Women should be allowed to choose whether to wait or to undergo induction immediately as the outcomes are the same.

D. Women with known GBS colonization should be recommended induction without delay.

E. Women induced with prostaglandin are less likely to need Syntocinon in labour.

*See Chapter 22, Pre-labour rupture of membranes.*

## 82. For women with preterm pre-labour rupture of membranes (PPROM):

A. Cervical length measurement is useful in predicting preterm labour.

B. The risk of placental abruption is approximately 5 per cent.

C. Single-course maternal steroid administration does not increase the risk of maternal infection.

D. Maternal steroid administration does not reduce the incidence of neonatal respiratory distress syndrome.

E. Antibiotic therapy improves neonatal mortality and morbidity rates.

*See Chapter 22, Pre-labour rupture of membranes.*

## 83. Planned induction of labour:

A. Should occur in less than 15 per cent of patients.

B. Should be performed before 41 weeks in cases of presumed fetal macrosomia.

C. In the presence of intact membranes, should involve prostaglandin administration regardless of the cervical status.

D. Should not be offered electively before 41 weeks' gestation.

E. Should not be offered to a patient who has previously been delivered by caesarean section.

*See Chapter 25, Induction of labour.*

## 84. Regarding induction of labour:

A. Uterine hyperstimuation secondary to prostaglandin administration is best treated with tocolysis.

B. Women with PROM at term (>37 weeks) should be offered a choice of immediate induction of labour or expectant management.

C. Uterine rupture occurs more frequently among women undergoing a trial of vaginal delivery following caesarean section in their previous pregnancy than among those undergoing elective repeat caesarean delivery.

D. Neonatal jaundice has been reported following the use of prostaglandins during induction of labour.

E. Women who do not labour after an induction should be offered caesarean section.

*See Chapter 25, Induction of labour.*

**85. Cephalo-pelvic disproportion (CPD) in the absence of gross pelvic abnormality can be diagnosed by:**

A. Ultrasound scan.

B. A maternal stature of less than 155 cm.

C. Lateral X-ray pelvimetry.

E. Pelvic examination.

F. Trial of vaginal delivery.

*See Chapter 27, Poor progress in labour.*

**86. Regarding progress in labour:**

A. A normal cervicometric curve is associated with a caesarean section rate of less than 5 per cent.

B. Primary dysfunctional labour occurs in 10 per cent of nulliparous labours.

C. In a case of secondary arrest, augmentation may be associated with uterine rupture.

D. A supportive partner during labour will reduce the incidence of delivery by caesarean section.

E. Augmentation with Syntocinon in the latent phase is associated with a reduction in the incidence of operative deliveries.

*See Chapter 27, Poor progress in labour.*

**87. With regard to electronic fetal monitoring:**

A. In low-risk pregnancies, continuous monitoring in labour has been shown to improve long-term outcomes.

B. An admission CTG should be performed for all women in labour.

C. Continuous fetal monitoring increases intervention in labour.

D. An abnormal CTG suggests acidosis in 50 per cent of fetuses.

E. Maternal oxygen therapy should be given if the CTG is pathological.

*See Chapter 29, Fetal compromise in the first stage of labour.*

**88. The following are normal in the first stage of labour:**

A. A scalp pH of 7.24.

B. A base excess of −13 mmol/L.

C. Baseline variability on the CTG of 5–10 bpm.

D. A baseline on CTG of 155 bpm.

E. Variable decelerations on CTG.

*See Chapter 29, Fetal compromise in the first stage of labour.*

**89. A classical caesarean section:**

A. Is performed through a midline sub-umbilical incision.

B. Has a higher incidence of postoperative pyrexia than a lower segment approach.

C. Is indicated in the presence of a placenta praevia at term.

D. Is the incision of choice in an HIV-positive woman.

*See Chapter 31, Caesarean section.*

**90.  Regarding caesarean section:**

A. It may be performed in a competent woman against her will for the benefit of the fetus.

B. The commonest indication for caesarean hysterectomy is uterine atony.

C. Vertical transmission of HIV may be reduced by 50 per cent.

D. The case fatality rate for all caesarean sections is eight times that for vaginal delivery.

*See Chapter 31, Caesarean section.*

**91.  Regarding fetal surveillance in the second stage of labour:**

A. Continuous electronic fetal monitoring is recommended.

B. There is no role for fetal blood sampling.

C. Ninety per cent of CTGs will show some abnormality.

D. Accelerations on CTG are commonly present.

E. Late decelerations are uncommon.

*See Chapter 32, Fetal compromise in the second stage of labour.*

**92.  The following increase the incidence of acidosis in the second stage of labour:**

A. Meconium staining of the liquor.

B. Active pushing.

C. Routine use of maternal oxygen therapy.

D. The absence of accelerations in an otherwise normal CTG.

E. Deep variable decelerations.

*See Chapter 32, Fetal compromise in the second stage of labour.*

**93.  Regarding shoulder dystocia:**

A. It affects approximately 1 per cent of all labours.

B. It carries a recurrence risk of 30 per cent.

C. It is commoner in obese women.

D. Twenty per cent of babies with an Erb's palsy will have long-term problems.

E. Erb's palsy can occur in babies delivered by caesarean section.

*See Chapter 33, Shoulder dystocia.*

**94.  The following manoeuvres are recommended for the management of shoulder dystocia:**

A. McRobert's.

B. Fundal pressure.

C. Suprapubic pressure.

D. Wood's screw.

E. Bilateral episiotomy.

*See Chapter 33, Shoulder dystocia.*

**95. The following have been shown to reduce the risk of second-degree perineal trauma in labour:**
A. Standing or squatting rather than lying prone.
B. Perineal massage in nulliparae.
C. Allowing spontaneous delivery of the head rather than controlling delivery.
D. Ventouse rather than forceps delivery.
E. Epidural analgesia.
   *See Chapter 36, Perineal trauma.*

**96. Perineal discomfort after delivery can be reduced by:**
A. Using a non-locking suture of the vaginal epithelium.
B. Using interrupted rather than subcuticular sutures to the perineal skin.
C. Using rapidly absorbable polyglactin sutures rather than standard polyglactin sutures.
D. Leaving the perineal skin approximated to within 0.5 cm but not closed.
E. Cleaning the episiotomy or trauma with saline rather than antiseptic.
   *See Chapter 36, Perineal trauma.*

**97. Regarding hypoxic–ischaemic encephalopathy (HIE):**
A. It affects approximately 1 per cent of infants.
B. Neurological sequelae are common in infants with mild HIE.
C. A persistently depressed Apgar score is associated with poor outcomes.
D. Most cases of cerebral palsy are due to HIE during labour.
E. Magnetic resonance imaging (MRI) is a useful modality in the first 48 hours of life.
F. Renal failure is commonly associated with severe HIE.
   *See Chapter 37, Perinatal asphyxia.*

**98. The following are features consistent with cerebral palsy secondary to an intrapartum event:**
A. Spastic diplegia.
B. A sentinel event during labour.
C. An Apgar score of 8 at 5 minutes.
D. A cord artery pH of 7.1.
E. Onset of fits at 24–48 hours of age.
   *See Chapter 37, Perinatal asphyxia.*

**99. Physiologically, the following are important considerations when resuscitating the newborn infant:**
A. The ductus arteriosus closes within hours of birth.
B. Pulmonary vascular pressures are increased by excessive use of high-concentration oxygen.
C. Hypothermia is associated with a worse neurological outcome.
D. Restoration of blood volume should be the priority to ensure adequate tissue perfusion.
E. Surfactant synthesis is affected by factors such as temperature, pH and hypoxaemia.
   *See Chapter 37, Perinatal asphyxia.*

**100.  At birth, the following are important:**
A. Oropharyngeal suction is the first priority to aid the infant to establish respiration.
B. History taking prior to birth is unnecessary as the principles of ABC (airways, breathing and circulation) apply regardless.
C. Preparation includes the checking of equipment, organization of staff, clear roles for individuals, good communication and parental involvement.
D. Catheterization of the umbilical vein requires a Seldinger technique as it is a central vessel.
E. Most neonatal resuscitation practice is based on well-researched evidence.
*See Chapter 37, Perinatal asphyxia.*

**101.  The Apgar score:**
A. Is an international scoring system used to help direct the resuscitation of a neonate.
B. Consists of five components, including heart rate, respiratory effort, skin colour, muscle tone and activity, and infant responsiveness.
C. Is very useful at predicting an infant's long-term outlook.
D. Is scored at 1 minute and 5 minutes after the birth of the whole child.
E. Is medico-legally an extremely important part of any resuscitation documentation.
*See Chapter 37, Perinatal asphyxia.*

**102.  During the resuscitation of an infant:**
A. The airway can be best maintained by placing the head in the neutral position.
B. The first steps involve drying the infant to maintain body warmth and stimulate the child to establish respiration.
C. Continual assessment of the infant's condition is mandatory.
D. Bag-valve-mask ventilation is performed at a rate of 30–40 inflations per minute, in contrast to ventilation via an endotracheal tube, which is performed at a rate of 60 breaths per minute.
E. Rescue breaths are more forceful, prolonged inflations used to help establish a functional residual volume in the lungs.
*See Chapter 37, Perinatal asphyxia.*

**103.  With regard to resuscitation in the newborn:**
A. Chest compressions at a rate of 120 per minute are more effectively achieved using the 'hands around the chest with the thumbs over the sternum' method as opposed to the use of two fingers placed over the sternum.
B. It is more important that the sternum is depressed a third of the antero-posterior diameter than that the rate of 120 compressions per minute is achieved when performing chest compressions.
C. The recommendation of high-concentration oxygen during resuscitation of the newborn is based on its associated protective effects on long-term lung damage.
D. Endotracheal adrenaline is as effective as intravascular adrenaline.
E. There is a medico-legal obligation to continue all resuscitative efforts for a minimum of 30 minutes without any signs of life before discontinuing care.
*See Chapter 38, Neonatal resuscitation.*

**104. When performing a newborn check, the following are important:**

A. The examination must be performed after 24 hours of life.

B. A clicky hip suggests a dislocated hip requiring orthopaedic management.

C. The Mongolian blue spot is a birthmark that is unimportant and can be ignored.

D. Discussion of an infant's feeding pattern with the mother should be a standard part of the newborn examination.

E. A neonate that has not opened its bowels by 24 hours of life needs to be investigated for possible Hirschprung's disease.

*See Chapter 37, Perinatal asphyxia.*

**105. The following increase the risk of GBS infection in the newborn infant:**

A. History of a previous infant with GBS infection.

B. Spontaneous onset of premature labour.

C. A positive urine culture for GBS in the mother during pregnancy.

D. Transient tachypnoea of the newborn following elective lower segment caesarean section.

E. Severe jaundice of the newborn presenting in the first 24 hours of life.

*See Chapter 37, Perinatal asphyxia.*

**106. These skin disorders are clinically significant in the newborn infant:**

A. Erythema toxicum neonatorum.

B. Traumatic cyanosis.

C. Aplasia cutis.

D. Flammeus naevus.

E. Miliaria.

*See Chapter 39, Common neonatal problems.*

**107. The following are true:**

A. Erb's palsy involving cervical nerve roots C3 and C4 is associated with a good outcome.

B. Hypothermia is associated with an increased risk of respiratory distress syndrome.

C. Cephalhaematomas that enlarge further at a few weeks of age indicate further bleeding and require investigation.

D. Sternomastoid tumours occur as a result of minor bleeding into the muscle and need physiotherapy to prevent shortening of the muscle as well as disturbance of visual development.

E. Fracture of the clavicle from birth requires immobilization of the arm for 48 hours.

*See Chapter 39, Common neonatal problems.*

**108. The following are commonly encountered in the newborn infant:**

A. Infants born at term by breech extraction are at high risk of hypoglycaemia if they have not fed within the first 2–4 hours.

B. Large bilateral hydroceles.

C. An innocent heart murmur as indicated by a soft thrill and radiation to the apex.

D. A deep-seated sacral dimple, the base of which is difficult to visualize.

E. Umbilical granulomas.

*See Chapter 39, Common neonatal problems.*

**109. Amniotic fluid embolism:**

A. Occurs in up to 1 in 2000 pregnancies.

B. Is the third commonest cause of direct maternal death in the UK.

C. Occurs most commonly immediately postpartum.

D. Is associated with artificial rupture of membranes.

*See Chapter 41, Postpartum collapse.*

**110. With regard to pulmonary embolism:**

A. It accounts for >50 per cent of all maternal deaths in the UK.

B. In pregnancy the risk is increased two-fold.

C. Antenatal presentation is most common.

D. It is associated with high body mass index.

*See Chapter 41, Postpartum collapse.*

**111. With regard to massive postpartum haemorrhage:**

A. It complicates 5 per cent of all pregnancies.

B. It is the third most common cause of direct maternal death in the UK.

C. Consumptive coagulopathy may worsen the prognosis.

D. If caused by uterine atony, it may be managed using a Rusch balloon.

*See Chapter 42, Postpartum haemorrhage.*

**112. Morbidly adherent and retained placenta:**

A. Is associated with elevated serum aFP.

B. Is associated with elevated serum βhCG.

C. Is more common in women under the age of 35 years.

D. Is more common in women who have placenta praevia.

*See Chapter 42, Postpartum haemorrhage.*

**113. In septic shock:**

A. Two to three per cent of pregnant women die.

B. The most common infective organisms in pregnancy are *Escherichia coli*.

C. Association with adult respiratory syndrome carries a mortality of 50 per cent.

D. There may be an association with systemic inflammatory response syndrome.

E. Administration of activated protein C may reduce mortality.

*See Chapter 43, Postpartum pyrexia.*

**114. Common causes of sepsis in obstetric cases include:**

A. Chorioamnionitis.

B. Intracerebral abscess.

C. Necrotizing fasciitis.

D. Pneumonia.

E. Pancreatitis.

*See Chapter 43, Postpartum pyrexia.*

**115. Adverse changes in postnatal affect:**

A. Occur in >50 per cent of women.

B. Are morbid in 25 per cent of women.

C. Are associated with psychosis in 5 per cent of women.

D. Are more common in women who have experienced them in a previous pregnancy.

*See Chapter 44, Disturbed mood.*

**116. With regard to postnatal depression:**

A. It may be associated with pre-conceptual psychiatric illness.

B. It may be controlled by adjuvant oestrogen therapy.

C. Tricyclic antidepressants are less effective than cognitive therapy.

D. It may be monitored using the Edinburgh Score.

*See Chapter 44, Disturbed mood.*

**117. Breastfeeding:**

A. Occurs in >50 per cent of pregnancies in the UK.

B. Is more common in women of lower socioeconomic class.

C. Is commonly performed for more than 12 months postnatally.

*See Chapter 45, Problems with breastfeeding.*

**118. Mastalgia:**

A. Is a common indication for cessation of breastfeeding.

B. Is associated with delayed neonatal feeding.

C. Has an increased incidence in mothers using supplementary feeding.

D. Is relieved by the use of anti-inflammatory agents.

*See Chapter 45, Problems with breastfeeding.*

# GYNAECOLOGY

**119. In the normal development of the female reproductive tract:**
A. The paramesonephric ducts develop at 10 weeks post-conception.
B. Anti-Müllerian hormone (AMH) leads to degeneration of the Müllerian ducts.
C. The paroophoron develops from the Wolffian ducts.
D. The myometrium develops from the Wolffian ducts.
E. The vaginal plate is derived from the urogenital sinus.
   *See Chapter 46, Normal and abnormal development of the genitalia.*

**120. Congenital adrenal hyperplasia:**
A. Presents classically as neonatal hypernatraemia.
B. Presents classically as a feminized XY neonate.
C. Causes absolute infertility.
D. Leads to high circulating concentrations of testosterone.
E. Requires mineralocorticoid replacement.
   *See Chapter 46, Normal and abnormal development of the genitalia.*

**121. The following statements refer to girls with congenital adrenal hyperplasia:**
A. The usual karyotype is 46XY.
B. Most cases are due to a deficiency of the 21-hydroxylase enzyme.
C. Müllerian structures fail to develop in utero.
D. Poor compliance with treatment leads to raised levels of 17-alpha hydroxyprogesterone.
E. Treated females have fertility rates that are similar to those of unaffected women.
   *See Chapter 47, Karyotypic abnormalities.*

**122. When compared to women with a normal karyotype, women with Turner's syndrome (45X) have an increased incidence of the following medical conditions:**
A. Ovarian carcinoma.
B. Hypertension.
C. Diabetes.
D. Cirrhosis of the liver.
E. Deafness.
   *See Chapter 47, Karyotypic abnormalities.*

### 123. Central precocious puberty:

A. Follows a premature suppression of pituitary luteinizing hormone (LH) and follicle-stimulating hormone (FSH) secretion due to activation of ovarian steroid synthesis.
B. Should be investigated with cranial imaging techniques.
C. Is frequently seen in girls with Turner's syndrome.
D. Is frequently accompanied by a cessation of growth.
E. Is frequently preceded by initiation of breast development.
*See Chapter 48, Menarche and adolescent gynaecology.*

### 124. In pubertal delay:

A. Elevated plasma concentrations of LH and FSH suggest a readily reversible cause.
B. A 45XO karyotype suggests that the uterus has not developed.
C. Steroids can be given to induce breast development.
D. Low concentrations of gonadotrophins are associated with excessive exercise.
E. Bone age is retarded in constitutional delayed puberty.
*See Chapter 48, Menarche and adolescent gynaecology.*

### 125. With regard to the human ovary:

A. The primordial follicles are embedded in the medulla.
B. The maximum size of the primordial follicle pool is attained at birth.
C. Ovulation does not occur in utero.
D. Similar to the testis, the ovary originates from a coelomic projection known as the gonadal ridge.
E. The hilar cells are differentiated cells that form the major source of ovarian peptide hormones.
*See Chapter 49, Ovarian and menstrual cycles.*

### 126. In an ovulatory cycle:

A. Usually only one follicle develops every cycle.
B. Both oestrogen and inhibin B are produced by the lead follicle.
C. Ovulation occurs 24–36 hours post-LH surge.
D. The LH triggers the completion of the first mitotic division, resulting in the production of the first polar body.
E. Follicular development is dependent on the gonadotrophins throughout the cycle.
*See Chapter 49, Ovarian and menstrual cycles.*

### 127. Condoms:

A. Have the additional benefit of reducing sexually transmitted diseases, including human immunodeficiency virus (HIV) disease.
B. Have a higher failure rate in circumcized men.
C. Have a reduced effectiveness in the presence of oestradiol creams.
D. Have a reduced effectiveness in the presence of K-Y jelly.
E. Have a quoted contraceptive efficacy of 3–23 per 100 woman-years.
*See Chapter 50, Contraception, sterilization and termination of pregnancy.*

**128. With regard to laparoscopic clip sterilization:**

A. There is a failure rate of approximately 0.5 per cent.

B. Most deaths are due to anaesthetic complications.

C. The procedure should not be performed during menstruation.

D. All women should be counselled that male sterilization is a safer alternative.

E. Surgical emphysema is a recognized complication.

*See Chapter 50, Contraception, sterilization and termination of pregnancy.*

**129. With regard to the normal menstrual cycle:**

A. The pulsatile release of gonadotrophin-releasing hormone (GnRH) increases in the luteal phase of the cycle.

B. The oestrogen surge precedes the LH surge by 12 hours.

C. Oestrogen receptor (ER) and progesterone receptor (PR) expression is maximal in the late luteal phase.

D. Ovulation occurs approximately 32 hours after the LH surge.

E. The number of endometrial leucocytes varies over the menstrual cycle.

*See Chapter 51.1, Endometrial function.*

**130. Uterine fibroids:**

A. Are present in up to 25 per cent of women of reproductive age.

B. Are the most common site of leiomyosarcoma development.

C. If small and submucous, are unlikely to be associated with menorrhagia.

D. Can be accurately located on pelvic ultrasound.

E. If palpable abdominally, should be removed.

*See Chapter 51.2, Uterine fibroids and menorrhagia.*

**131. Recognized side effects of danazol include:**

A. Weight gain.

B. Vaginal dryness.

C. Increase in breast size.

D. Acne.

E. Hirsutism.

*See Chapter 51.2, Uterine fibroids and menorrhagia.*

**132. In the management of menorrhagia:**

A. Norethisterone is the treatment of choice for reducing menstrual loss in simple menorrhagia.

B. Oestrogen-impregnated intrauterine devices are useful for reducing menstrual loss.

C. Hysteroscopy allows visualization of the ovarian surfaces.

D. Endometrial sampling on day 7 of the cycle will usually reveal proliferative endometrium.

E. GnRH agonists are a cost-effective alternative to the oral contraceptive pill.

*See Chapter 51.3, Heavy and irregular menstruation.*

### 133. The following relate to dysmenorrhoea:

A. Childbirth has a curative effect on secondary dysmenorrhoea.
B. Women who have smoked for more than 10 years have an increased risk of dysmenorrhoea.
C. Pain prior to menstruation suggests pelvic inflammatory disease (PID).
D. In secondary dysmenorrhoea, laparoscopy should be considered if a trial of therapy is unsuccessful.
E. The contraceptive pill is of value in its treatment.

*See Chapter 51.4, Dysmenorrhoea.*

### 134. With regard to endometriosis:

A. It is associated with unruptured luteinized follicle.
B. The severity of disease is determined by the American Fertility Score.
C. It can be treated with 200 mg danazol daily.
D. The results of medical treatment are poor compared to those of surgery.
E. It cannot occur de novo after sterilization.

*See Chapter 51.5, Endometriosis and gonadotrophin releasing hormone analogues.*

### 135. The diagnosis of adenomyosis requires:

A. A myometrial thickness of 2.5 cm or more.
B. Islands of endometrial glands without stroma in the myometrium.
C. Accompanying endometriosis elsewhere in the pelvis.
D. Extension of the endometrial glands and stroma in the myometrium with adjacent smooth muscle hyperplasia.
E. Subserosal disease near the uterine surface.

*See Chapter 51.6, Adenomyosis.*

### 136. With regard to premenstrual syndrome:

A. It is a common clinical phenomenon affecting 40 per cent of the female population.
B. The symptoms occur at a time of relative progesterone deficiency.
C. It is not relieved by the end of menstruation.
D. Evening primrose oil is effective at relieving the symptoms.
E. Suppression of ovulation with transdermal oestrogen and progesterone for endometrial protection is an effective treatment.

*See Chapter 51.7, Premenstrual syndrome.*

### 137. When investigating an infertile couple:

A. Routine hysteroscopy should be carried out.
B. A serum progesterone level >10 nmol/L on cycle day 21 is indicative of ovulation.
C. Laparoscopy and dye hydrotubation is more informative of uterine cavity abnormality than hysterosalpingography.
D. Urinary LH detection using a commercially available test kit is diagnostic of ovulation.
E. A routine cervical smear should be included in the investigation of infertility.

*See Chapter 52.2, Female infertility.*

### 138. In the management of female infertility:

A. Three cycles of superovulation and intrauterine insemination result in a better pregnancy rate compared to one in-vitro fertilization (IVF) cycle in patients with unexplained infertility.

B. Ectopic pregnancy rates are similar between IVF and gamete intrafallopian transfer (GIFT) in patients with unexplained infertility.

C. Tubal surgery for hydrosalpynx results in pregnancy in more than 50 per cent of cases.

D. Infertile patients with mild endometriosis should be given long-term GnRH agonist treatment while awaiting IVF treatment.

E. Salpingectomy in patients with tubal factor infertility undergoing IVF improves the pregnancy rates.

*See Chapter 52.2, Female infertility.*

### 139. Regarding male factor investigations:

A. Semen analysis should be performed before investigations of the female partner.

B. Testing for anti-sperm antibodies should be carried out routinely.

C. The ratio of normal to abnormal sperm morphology is a sensitive marker of male fertility.

D. Testicular examination is ideally carried out in the supine position.

E. Ten per cent of azoospermic and severely oligozoospermic men are carriers of the cystic fibrosis gene.

*See Chapter 52.3, Male infertility.*

### 140. Regarding the management of male factor infertility:

A. Varicocelectomy is effective in improving male fertility when associated with severe oligospermia.

B. Bromocriptine is useful in treating sperm abnormalities and sexual dysfunction in infertile men.

C. Patients with Kallmann's syndrome can be treated effectively with gonadotrophins.

D. Sperm washing and intrauterine insemination are effective in treating asthenospermia due to anti-sperm antibodies.

E. Obtaining and freezing a sperm sample from the epididymis is essential during vasectomy reversal as the procedure has a high failure rate.

*See Chapter 52.3, Male infertility.*

### 141. The following statements are true:

A. IVF is a suitable first-line option for treating all types of infertility.

B. Optional transfer of two instead of three embryos does not reduce the pregnancy rate.

C. Transferring two or three embryos has the same twin pregnancy rates.

D. Not proceeding with embryo transfer prevents late-onset ovarian hyperstimulation syndrome (OHSS).

E. Recombinant FSH offers a higher pregnancy rate compared to high-purity urinary gonadotrophins.

*See Chapter 52.4, Assisted reproduction.*

### 142. With regard to OHSS:

A. It can lead to hypovolaemia and haemoconcentration in severe cases.
B. Mild and moderate cases can be treated at home.
C. Albumin replacement is essential for most cases.
D. Paracentesis should be avoided at all costs.
E. It is commoner in polycystic ovarian syndrome (PCOS) and lean patients.
   *See Chapter 52.4, Assisted reproduction.*

### 143. Polycystic ovarian syndrome:

A. Is associated with LH hypersecretion.
B. Is associated with low TSH levels.
C. Typically presents with primary amenorrhoea.
D. Is associated with increased production of dehydroepiandrosterone sulphate (DHEAS), an adrenal androgen.
E. Is associated with markedly elevated serum prolactin.
   *See Chapter 53, Polycystic ovarian syndrome.*

### 144. The following are inconsistent with a diagnosis of PCOS:

A. A regular 28-day cycle.
B. Normal ovarian morphology on ultrasound scan.
C. LH:FSH ratio <2:1.
D. Normal body mass index.
E. Rapidly progressive virilization.
   *See Chapter 53, Polycystic ovarian syndrome.*

### 145. With respect to the management of anovulatory infertility in a woman with PCOS:

A. Weight reduction is ineffective in improving fertility.
B. Ultrasound follicular tracking is not necessary if clomiphene citrate is used for fewer than 12 cycles.
C. Use of clomiphene citrate for fewer than 12 cycles has been shown to be associated with an increased risk of ovarian cancer.
D. Tamoxifen is an alternative to clomiphene citrate.
E. The recommended duration of use of gonadotrophin therapy is 6–12 months.
   *See Chapter 53, Polycystic ovarian syndrome.*

### 146. With respect to the management of anovulatory infertility in a woman PCOS:

A. Laparoscopic ovarian drilling is more effective than gonadotrophin therapy in women who are clomiphene resistant.
B. Laparoscopic ovarian drilling is associated with an increased risk of multiple pregnancy.
C. Laparoscopic ovarian drilling is associated with OHSS.
D. Ultrasound follicular tracking is unnecessary in women treated with laparoscopic ovarian drilling.
E. Laparoscopic ovarian drilling is associated with a normalization of LH levels.
   *See Chapter 53, Polycystic ovarian syndrome.*

**147. The following are long-term consequences of PCOS:**

A. Increased mortality from cardiovascular disease.

B. Increased risk of ovarian cancer.

C. Increased risk of endometrial cancer.

D. Increased risk of insulin-dependent diabetes mellitus.

E. Increased risk of osteoporosis.

*See Chapter 53, Polycystic ovarian syndrome.*

**148. PCOS is associated with:**

A. Increased levels of sex hormone-binding globulin (SHBG).

B. Increased ovarian production of DHEAS.

C. Increased ovarian production of androstenedione.

D. Increased ovarian production of testosterone.

E. Unopposed oestrogenic stimulation of the endometrium.

*See Chapter 53, Polycystic ovarian syndrome.*

**149. With respect to androgen production in the female:**

A. Testosterone is the main adrenal androgen.

B. Androstenedione is the main ovarian androgen.

C. Androstenedione and DHEA do not have androgenic activity.

D. DHEAS is almost exclusively of adrenal origin.

E. Androstenedione and DHEA are converted to testosterone in peripheral tissues.

*See Chapter 54, Hirsutism and virilism.*

**150. When a 30-year-old woman presents with rapidly progressive hirsutism and virilization:**

A. Ovarian hilus cell tumour is a possible diagnosis.

B. Ovarian granulosa theca cell tumour is a likely diagnosis.

C. A tumour of the adrenal medulla is a possible cause.

D. Excision of an androgen-producing ovarian tumour results in a rapid regression of hirsutism.

E. PCOS is a possible diagnosis.

*See Chapter 54, Hirsutism and virilism.*

**151. The following drugs are associated with hirsutism:**

A. Danazol.

B. Phenytoin.

C. Cyclosporin A.

D. Norethisterone.

E. Finasteride.

*See Chapter 54, Hirsutism and virilism.*

**152. With respect to drug treatment for hirsutism:**

A. The combined oral contraceptive pill (COCP) reduces SHBG production.

B. Medroxyprogesterone acetate reduces LH production.

C. Progestogens inhibit 5-alpha reductase activity.

D. Flutamide is a 5-alpha reductase inhibitor.

E. Finasteride is a testosterone antagonist.

*See Chapter 54, Hirsutism and virilism.*

**153. The following syndromes are typically associated with primary amenorrhoea:**

A. Rokitansky's syndrome.

B. Turner's syndrome.

C. Sheehan's syndrome.

D. Kallmann's syndrome.

E. Asherman's syndrome.

*See Chapter 55, Amenorrhoea and oligomenorrhoea.*

**154. The following are likely diagnoses in a 16-year-old female with primary amenorrhoea but normal development of the breasts and external genitalia.**

A. Turner's syndrome.

B. Complete androgen insensitivity syndrome.

C. Uterine agenesis.

D. Kallmann's syndrome.

E. Hyperprolactinaemia.

*See Chapter 55, Amenorrhoea and oligomenorrhoea.*

**155. Gonadectomy is indicated because of the risk of malignancy in women with primary amenorrhoea and the following conditions:**

A. Turner's syndrome.

B. Androgen insensitivity syndrome.

C. Gonadal dysgenesis with 46XY karyotype.

D. Gonadal dysgenesis with 46XX karyotype.

E. Rokitansky's syndrome.

*See Chapter 55, Amenorrhoea and oligomenorrhoea.*

**156. The following diagnoses are likely in a 30-year-old woman with secondary amenorrhoea and low gonadotrophin levels:**

A. Premature ovarian failure.

B. Resistant ovary syndrome.

C. Sheehan's syndrome.

D. Asherman's syndrome.

E. Post-pill amenorrhoea.

*See Chapter 55, Amenorrhoea and oligomenorrhoea.*

**157. Regarding the menopause:**

A. In the Western world between 70 and 80 per cent of women going through the menopause experience hot flushes.

B. Most oral oestrogens lead to an increase in high-density lipoprotein (HDL) cholesterol and a fall in low-density lipoprotein (LDL) cholesterol.

C. Women with a fractured neck of femur have a 40 per cent chance of dying within a year.

D. Alzheimer's disease accounts for more than 50 per cent of all cases of dementia.

E. All women receiving hormone replacement therapy (HRT) should have a pelvic and breast examination, their weight should be measured, and blood taken for electrolyte and lipid levels before commencing therapy.

*See Chapter 56, Menopause and hormone replacement therapy.*

**158. Regarding treatment of the menopause:**

A. Double-blind studies have shown clonidine to be effective in the treatment of hot flushes and night sweats.

B. Continuous combined preparations are more effective than sequential preparations at preventing endometrial cancer.

C. Progestogenic side effects include bloating, mastalgia, fluid retention and acne.

D. Fifty per cent of women discontinue HRT within 3 years of starting treatment.

E. Patients with breast cancer should never receive HRT.

*See Chapter 56, Menopause and hormone replacement therapy.*

**159. In the management of bleeding in early pregnancy:**

A. The beta subunit of human chorionic gonadotrophin (βhCG) measured in maternal blood originates from the fetus.

B. At 7 weeks' gestation, an observed increase of βhCG from 1500 to 2000 IU/ml over 48 hours is likely to indicate the presence of an early viable intrauterine pregnancy.

C. An unruptured tubal ectopic pregnancy in a 22-year-old nulliparous woman with previous unilateral salpingectomy is best treated with salpingectomy.

D. Methotrexate treatment of an unruptured tubal ectopic pregnancy results in a prompt fall in concentrations of βhCG measured in maternal blood.

E. In the days following methotrexate treatment, patients should be advised to avoid the use of non-steroidal anti-inflammatory drugs (NSAIDs).

*See Chapter 57, Problems in early pregnancy.*

**160. Following complete miscarriage of a first pregnancy at 6 weeks' gestation:**

A. Attempts to conceive again should be avoided for three menstrual cycles.

B. Failure to give anti-D to Rhesus (Rh)-negative patients is likely to lead to Rh sensitization in a subsequent pregnancy.

C. The risk of miscarriage of the second pregnancy is approximately 25 per cent.

D. Diagnosis should be confirmed by dilatation and curettage.

E. The couple should be offered a thrombophilia screen.

*See Chapter 57, Problems in early pregnancy.*

**161. With regard to urinary tract infections (UTIs):**
A. Overall, 5 per cent of women have asymptomatic bacteriuria.
B. Thirty per cent of women will develop a UTI in their lifetime.
C. *Escherichia coli* is the main causative organism.
D. Recurrent UTIs are rarely caused by the same organism.
E. Urethral catheters are associated with higher rates of infection than suprapubic catheters.
   *See Chapter 61, Lower urinary tract infections.*

**162. Considering the treatment of urinary tract infections:**
A. Bacteriuria should usually be treated.
B. Bacteriuria should usually be treated in pregnancy.
C. Cranberry juice has been proven to be effective.
D. Amoxycillin is effective as a single-dose agent.
E. Vaginal oestrogens are effective in the management of postmenopausal women with recurrent UTIs.
   *See Chapter 61, Lower urinary tract infections.*

**163. Urogenital prolapse:**
A. Accounts for 50 per cent of all gynaecological procedures.
B. Rarely occurs in nulliparous women.
C. May be associated with lower urinary tract symptoms.
D. Is more common following the menopause.
E. Is found in 30 per cent of elderly women.
   *See Chapter 62, Urogenital prolapse.*

**164. With regard to the management of urogenital prolapse:**
A. Physiotherapy has been shown to be effective.
B. Ring pessaries are the management of choice in the elderly.
C. Sacrospinous ligament fixation should be performed routinely at vaginal hysterectomy to prevent vault prolapse.
D. Enterocele formation is increased following colposuspension.
E. Anterior repair is an effective treatment for co-existent stress incontinence.
   *See Chapter 62, Urogenital prolapse.*

**165. The following investigations are useful in women suspected of having PID:**
A. Pregnancy test.
B. Endocervical test for *Chlamydia trachomatis*.
C. Endocervical test for *Neisseria gonorrhoeae*.
D. Erythrocyte sedimentation rate (ESR).
E. Carcinoembryonic antigen (CEA).
F. Plain abdominal X-ray.
   *See Chapter 63.1, Infection and sexual health.*

**166. The following are signs and symptoms of PID:**
A. Lower abdominal pain.
B. Dyspareunia.
C. Menorrhagia as a new symptom.
D. Abnormal vaginal discharge.
E. Cervical excitation.
F. Right upper quadrant discomfort.
G. Breakthrough bleeding on the COCP.
*See Chapter 63.1, Infection and sexual health.*

**167. *Chlamydia trachomatis*:**
A. Is diagnosed by culture of cervical purulent discharge.
B. Has been found to be carried by an increased number of women using the COCP.
C. Is usually symptomatic.
D. Is routinely treated with penicillins.
*See Chapter 63.1, Infection and sexual health.*

**168. With regard to genital herpes simplex infection in pregnancy:**
A. Aciclovir is not used.
B. Vaginal delivery would be anticipated except for those developing symptoms of a first episode after 34 weeks' gestation.
C. Continuous antiviral therapy is indicated in the last 4 weeks of pregnancy in those who have a first episode of infection in the first and second trimesters of pregnancy.
D. It is diagnosed by high vaginal swab.
*See Chapter 63.1, Infection and sexual health.*

**169. Dyspareunia is associated with:**
A. Vaginal infection.
B. Allergic dermatitis of the vulva.
C. Involuntary spasm of the pubo-coccygeal muscles.
D. Poor sexual technique.
E. Urinary tract infection.
*See Chapter 63.2, Dyspareunia and other psychosexual problems.*

**170. With regard to sexual history taking:**
A. Gynaecologists do not need to be comfortable to talk about sexual intercourse in detail.
B. The age of the adult patient should determine whether sex is mentioned during the consultation.
C. Talking about sex prior to gynaecological surgery is not appropriate.
*See Chapter 63.2, Dyspareunia and other psychosexual problems.*

**171.  Child sex abuse:**

A. Cannot take place in children under 3 years of age.

B. Includes exposure.

C. Can be managed solely by the gynaecologist who diagnoses the problem.

D. Can be diagnosed confidently after discovering that a 13-year-old is not *virgo intacta*.

   *See Chapter 63.3, Child sex abuse.*

**172.  The following may be adult sequelae of child sex abuse:**

A. Persistent vaginal discharge.

B. Anxiety disorders.

C. Promiscuity.

D. Alcohol abuse.

   *See Chapter 63.3, Child sex abuse.*

**173.  With regard to the management of rape victims:**

A. The timing of the examination is not relevant.

B. Forensic sampling is the priority of the examination.

C. Informed consent should be obtained prior to the forensic medical examination.

D. Clothing should not be sent for forensic examination.

E. Screening for sexually transmitted diseases should be offered to the victim.

   *See Chapter 63.4, Rape and rape counselling.*

**174.  With regard to rape:**

A. It is defined as 'unlawful sexual intercourse by a woman with a man, by force, fear or fraud'.

B. Rape victims should be examined by specialist forensic medical examiners.

C. Fifty per cent of rape victims have major non-genital injuries.

D. Genital photographs should be taken by a photographer of a different gender.

E. Post-exposure HIV prophylaxis should be continued for 3 months.

   *See Chapter 63.4, Rape and rape counselling.*

**175.  With regard to vulval lichen sclerosus:**

A. Histological diagnosis is mandatory.

B. Emollient creams are ineffective.

C. Eighty per cent of cases will respond to 1% hydrocortisone cream.

D. Testosterone cream is useful for maintaining response.

E. The condition is usually self-limiting.

   *See Chapter 64, Benign vulval problems.*

**176. With regard to vulval skin diseases:**

A. Seborrhoeic dermatitis is a fungal condition.

B. Hidradenitis suppurativa is a disorder of the eccrine glands.

C. Psoriasis affecting the vulva is best managed with tar preparations.

D. In vulvovaginal candidiasis, topical antifungals are less effective than oral preparations.

E. Lichen planus is a pre-malignant condition.

*See Chapter 64, Benign vulval problems.*

**177. In vulval vestibulitis:**

A. Pain is occasionally associated with light touch in the vestibule area.

B. Vestibular erythema is necessary to make a diagnosis.

C. The modified vestibulectomy produces a success rate of 70 per cent in well-selected patients.

D. Sensate focus therapy should complement the physical treatments among those patients with sexual dysfunction.

E. Amitryptyline is the first-line treatment of choice.

*See Chapter 65, Vulval pain syndromes.*

**178. In dysaesthetic vulvodynia:**

A. The pain experienced by the patient is typically neuropathic.

B. Patients are usually 20–30 years of age.

C. The standard dosage of amitryptyline is 10 mg/day.

D. Irritant contact dermatitis of the vulva can occur.

E. Peri-anal pain may also occur.

*See Chapter 65, Vulval pain syndromes.*

**179. With regard to human papillomaviruses (HPVs):**

A. They are RNA viruses of about 8000 base pairs.

B. HPV 16 is the commonest oncogenic genital type.

C. Different types can be distinguished by electron microscopy.

D. The prevalence of genital HPV infection decreases with advancing age.

E. The host's main response to infection is antibody mediated.

*See Chapter 66, Pre-invasive disease.*

**180. With regard to the National Health Service (NHS) cervical screening programme:**

A. Since organized screening was introduced, there has been a fall in the incidence of cervical cancer.

B. More than 80 per cent of eligible women are covered by the programme.

C. About 25 per cent of smears are reported as 'not normal'.

D. Women are screened with a maximum 3-yearly cycle.

E. General practitioners are paid according to whether they meet coverage targets for cervical smears.

*See Chapter 66, Pre-invasive disease.*

**181. In the investigation of postmenopausal bleeding:**
A. Transvaginal ultrasound scanning (TVUS) has a high sensitivity.
B. Magnetic resonance imaging (MRI) should be used if available.
C. Endometrial biopsy is often necessary.
D. Outpatient hysteroscopy is the investigation of choice.
E. Pelvic examination can be replaced by TVUS.
*See Chapter 67, Endometrial cancer.*

**182. Following surgery for endometrial cancer:**
A. Vault brachytherapy will improve survival.
B. HRT is contraindicated.
C. Pelvic irradiation will reduce the risk of pelvic recurrence.
D. Tamoxifen for a previous breast cancer may be continued.
E. Adjuvant progesterone therapy is not usually of benefit.
*See Chapter 67, Endometrial cancer.*

**183. With regard to micro-invasive disease:**
A. It is associated with nodal disease in 20 per cent of cases.
B. It can be cured by large loop excision of the transformation zone (LLETZ).
C. It is associated with a depth of invasion of 9 mm.
D. It always requires radical hysterectomy.
E. Pelvic lymphadenectomy should only be performed in selected cases.
*See Chapter 68, Cervical cancer.*

**184. With regard to stage Ib cervical cancer:**
A. Squamous carcinoma is the most common type.
B. Small-cell type is associated with distant metastases.
C. It can be treated by chemoradiotherapy.
D. Following surgery, disease-free vaginal margins of <5 mm should be considered for adjuvant chemotherapy.
E. Radical surgery is associated with chronic voiding problems.
*See Chapter 68, Cervical cancer.*

**185. In the treatment of ovarian cancer:**
A. Standard adjuvant therapy involves intravenous chemotherapy.
B. Adjuvant therapy is not indicated for patients with stage Ic disease.
C. Paclitaxel and carboplatin are prescribed for patients with advanced disease.
D. Alkylating agents are the mainstay of treatment.
E. Response rates to second-line chemotherapy are of the order of 70 per cent.
*See Chapter 69, Benign and malignant ovarian masses.*

**186. Malignant germ-cell tumours:**

A. Account for 15 per cent of all ovarian malignancies.

B. Represent 60 per cent of ovarian cancers in children and adolescents.

C. Are usually bilateral.

D. Have an overall 5-year survival rate of 38 per cent.

E. Require treatment that usually results in infertility.

*See Chapter 69, Benign and malignant ovarian masses.*


**187. With regard to cancer of the vulva:**

A. It is linked to HPV in 90 per cent of all cases.

B. It develops in 4 per cent of cases of lichen sclerosus.

C. It develops in 80 per cent of cases of treated vulval intraepithelial neoplasia 3 (VIN3).

D. Melanoma of the vulva is the second most common type.

E. It most commonly affects the perineum.

*See Chapter 70, Vulval and vaginal cancer.*


**188. In the treatment of vulval cancer:**

A. All stage I vulval cancers require a bilateral inguinal lymph node dissection.

B. Superficial inguinal node dissection has the same rate of groin recurrence as an inguino-femoral node dissection.

C. The risk of recurrence following surgery for stage I/II disease is the same for a triple incision technique and an 'en-bloc' radical vulvectomy.

D. Adjuvant radiotherapy is recommended when there is extracapsular lymph node spread in a single lymph node.

E. Chemoradiotherapy has a cure rate equivalent to that of surgery in the treatment of stage II vulva cancer.

*See Chapter 70, Vulval and vaginal cancer.*


**189. Complete hydatidiform moles:**

A. Are usually diploid.

B. Give rise to persistent trophoblastic disease in 50 per cent of cases.

C. Can co-exist with a normal 'twin' conceptus.

D. Usually present after the 16th week of pregnancy.

E. Are commonly repetitive.

*See Chapter 71, Gestational trophoblastic disease.*


**190. Partial hydatidiform moles:**

A. Are usually triploid.

B. Rarely give rise to persistent trophoblastic disease.

C. Often present as a missed miscarriage.

D. Are easy to diagnose on ultrasound scan.

E. Often have recognizable embryonic and fetal tissues.

*See Chapter 71, Gestational trophoblastic disease.*

# OBSTETRICS

### 1. In chronic hypertension in pregnancy:

A. The perinatal risk is only increased in the presence of proteinuria. **False**

B. The use of thiazide diuretics is associated with teratogenesis. **False**

C. First trimester use of angiotensin-converting enzyme (ACE) inhibitors is an indication for a termination of pregnancy. **False**

D. Methyldopa is free of side effects. **False**

E. The relative risk of pre-eclampsia supervening is more than doubled. **True**

Fetal growth restriction and abruptio placentae occur more frequently in isolated chronic hypertension (in the absence of proteinuria). Although thiazide diuretics are contraindicated as they reduce plasma volume, they are not associated with teratogenesis. Neonatal thrombocytopenia has also been reported with the use of thiazide diuretics in pregnancy. ACE inhibitors can lead to fetal renal compromise, but if stopped in early pregnancy the effects are usually reversible. Methyldopa can cause depression and tiredness and, very occasionally, liver dysfunction. The risk of pre-eclampsia is dependent on the level of blood pressure in early pregnancy, and has been reported to be as high as 20 per cent.

*See Chapter 6.1, Chronic hypertension.*

### 2. When treating moderate hypertension in pregnancy:

A. The risk of pre-eclampsia is reduced. **False**

B. The risk of severe hypertension is reduced. **True**

C. There is an increase in birth weight. **False**

D. Calcium channel blockers are contraindicated as they have tocolytic effects. **False**

E. Treatment should be discontinued 24 hours after delivery. **False**

There is no evidence that anti-hypertensive therapy alters the risk of getting pre-eclampsia. The only benefit shown in the meta-analysis of anti-hypertensive treatment is a significant reduction in the incidence of severe hypertension. There is a reported association between treatment and a reduction in birth weight. Calcium channel blockers such as nifedipine are frequently used, particularly as second-line treatment, and have negligible tocolytic effect. Blood pressure is frequently highest after 24 hours postpartum. Treatment should therefore be continued immediately postpartum.

*See Chapter 6.1, Chronic hypertension.*

### 3.  With regard to chronic hypertension:

| | |
|---|---|
| A. It affects 0.1 per cent of pregnant women. | **False** |
| B. ACE inhibitors are associated with fetal renal failure. | **True** |
| C. Labetolol is associated with intrauterine growth restriction (IUGR). | **True** |
| D. Fifty per cent of affected women will develop superimposed pre-eclampsia. | **False** |
| E. The second most common complication is placental abruption. | **True** |

Chronic hypertension is a common disease encountered in pregnancy and affects 1–2 per cent of pregnant women. ACE inhibitors are associated with fetal anuria, renal failure and hypocalvaria. However, importantly, the risks associated with ACE inhibitors are restricted to their use in the second and third trimesters. Therefore, these drugs should be discontinued as soon as pregnancy is diagnosed. Although labetolol, nifedipine and methyldopa are all drugs that can be used safely in pregnancy, they are associated with various side effects. Labetolol has been associated with IUGR, neonatal hypoglycaemia and fetal and neonatal bradycardias. Methyldopa is a centrally acting alpha-receptor agonist that is associated with maternal depression. Twenty per cent of women with chronic hypertension will develop superimposed pre-eclampsia during pregnancy. The second most common complication of chronic hypertension is placental abruption, with a rate of between 2 and 10 per cent.

*See Chapter 6.1, Chronic hypertension.*

### 4.  With regard to the management of diabetes mellitus in pregnancy:

| | |
|---|---|
| A. Frequent umbilical Doppler velocimetry will reduce the perinatal mortality rate. | **False** |
| B. A rise in insulin requirements at term is a poor prognostic sign. | **False** |
| C. Caesarean section is indicated if the estimated fetal weight is >3.5 kg. | **False** |
| D. Polyhydramnios can be prevented by insulin therapy. | **False** |

The value of umbilical artery Doppler in the monitoring of diabetic pregnancies is questionable. Insulin requirements increase in the second and third trimesters; it has been suggested that where insulin requirements suddenly fall, careful consideration must be given to delivery, as this may be suggestive of a 'failing' placenta. Even when the control is good, the incidence of polyhydramnios in diabetes is 5–13 per cent. One advocated strategy is to counsel regarding elective caesarean delivery when the estimated fetal weight is 4.5 kg or more. When the estimated fetal weight is between 4.0 and 4.5 kg, additional factors such as the past obstetric history should be taken into consideration.

*See Chapter 6.2, Diabetes mellitus.*

## 5. With regard to diabetes mellitus:

A. It complicates 1–2 per cent of pregnancies in the UK.                                    **True**

B. The complication of diabetic ketoacidosis is associated with a 50 per cent fetal
mortality rate.                                                                              **True**

C. A maternal four-dose insulin regimen gives better maternal and fetal outcomes
than a two-dose regimen.                                                                     **True**

D. In poorly controlled women the risk of fetal polyhydramnios is 25–30 per cent.           **True**

E. The congenital malformation rate is five to ten times that of non-diabetic
pregnancies.                                                                                 **True**

Diabetes is a common maternal condition that complicates pregnancy. The overall incidence
in the UK is 1–2 per cent; however, there is great geographical and ethnic diversity. The
congenital malformation rate is five to ten times higher than for non-diabetic pregnancies;
these malformations characteristically affect the central nervous, cardiovascular, skeletal,
gastrointestinal and genitourinary systems.

*See Chapter 6.2, Diabetes mellitus.*

## 6. The infant of a diabetic mother is at increased risk of:

A. Polycythaemia.                                                                            **True**

B. Hypermagnesaemia.                                                                         **False**

C. Traumatic delivery.                                                                       **True**

D. Neonatal jaundice.                                                                        **True**

E. Hypoglycaemia.                                                                            **True**

The infant of a diabetic mother is at increased risk of various metabolic and traumatic insults.
The fetus is at increased risk of hypogylcaemia, hypocalcaemia and hypomagnesaemia.

*See Chapter 6.2, Diabetes mellitus.*

### 7. The following conditions are contraindications to pregnancy:

| | |
|---|---|
| A. Wolf–Parkinson–White syndrome. | **False** |
| B. Eisenmenger's syndrome. | **True** |
| C. Mild mitral stenosis. | **False** |
| D. Primary pulmonary hypertension. | **True** |
| E. Marfan's syndrome with a dilated aortic root. | **True** |

Wolf–Parkinson–White syndrome causes supraventricular tachycardias due to an accessory pathway. Women may require maintenance anti-dysrhythmics, and acute episodes of supraventricular tachycardia may be treated with adenosine in pregnancy. Pregnancy is not contraindicated. Eisenmenger's syndrome is associated with a 40 per cent maternal mortality. In the event of a woman declining therapeutic termination of pregnancy, management is with elective admission in mid-pregnancy for oxygen, bed rest and thromboprophylaxis. The risk of pulmonary oedema in mitral stenosis is related to the severity of the stenosis. Mild mitral stenosis is usually well tolerated but requires close monitoring. Pulmonary hypertension from *any* cause is associated with a high maternal mortality. Management is as for Eisenmenger's syndrome. The risk of aortic dissection or rupture is increased in Marfan's syndrome and particularly in those whose aortic root is dilated prior to pregnancy or shows progressive dilatation during pregnancy. Women with aortic roots >4–4.5 cm should be advised to delay pregnancy until after aortic root repair.

*See Chapter 6.3, Cardiac disease.*

### 8. With regard to peripartum cardiomyopathy:

| | |
|---|---|
| A. It occurs in the last month of pregnancy. | **True** |
| B. Risk factors include multiple pregnancy, hypertension and nulliparity. | **False** |
| C. Cardiac transplantation is inappropriate. | **False** |
| D. Anticoagulation is required. | **True** |
| E. Cerebral embolization is a major cause of morbidity. | **True** |

Peripartum cardiomyopathy occurs late in pregnancy and can occur up to 5 months after delivery. Risk factors for this pathology include multiple pregnancy, hypertension, multiparity and increased age.

*See Chapter 6.3, Cardiac disease.*

## 9. Pregnancy is associated with:

| | |
|---|---|
| A. Increased thyroid-binding globulin. | **True** |
| B. Increased free thyroxine (T4). | **False** |
| C. Increased free triiodothyronine (T3). | **False** |
| D. Decreased maternal iodide levels. | **True** |
| E. Increased total T4. | **True** |

Thyroid-binding globulin increases in the first 2 weeks of pregnancy, and reaches a plateau by 20 weeks' gestation. This increase leads to an increase in the serum concentrations of total T4 and T3, but there are no changes in the amount of free circulating (unbound) thyroid hormones. There is iodine deficiency in pregnancy as a result of loss through increased glomerular filtration; fetal thyroid activity also depletes the maternal iodide pool.

*See Chapter 6.4, Thyroid disease.*

## 10. Propylthiouracil (PTU) therapy for a pregnant woman with Graves' disease:

| | |
|---|---|
| A. Reduces the titre of thyroid-stimulating hormone (TSH) receptor antibodies. | **True** |
| B. Inhibits the peripheral conversion of T3 to T4. | **False** |
| C. Is associated with teratogenesis. | **False** |
| D. Can cause agranulocytosis. | **True** |

Propylthiouracil reduces the titre of TSH receptor antibodies, and directly influences the pathogenesis of Graves' disease. It inhibits T4 synthesis by blocking the incorporation of iodine into tyrosine, and also inhibits the peripheral conversion of T4 to T3. Although PTU crosses the placenta, it is not thought to be teratogenic. Antithyroid drugs can cause agranulocytosis, and so a sore throat should be thoroughly investigated.

*See Chapter 6.4, Thyroid disease.*

## 11. Untreated hypothyroidism in pregnancy is associated with:

| | |
|---|---|
| A. Weight gain, hyperactivity, tachycardia. | **False** |
| B. Increased rate of miscarriage, pre-eclampsia and low-birth-weight babies. | **True** |
| C. An increased risk of congenital anomalies. | **False** |
| D. Reduced intelligence quotient (IQ) in infants. | **True** |
| E. Delayed infant neurodevelopment. | **True** |

Maternal hypothyroid complicates approximately 1 per cent of pregnancies. The clinical symptoms include weight gain, lethargy, hair loss, constipation, slow pulse and delayed relaxation of reflexes. In most cases it occurs through autoimmune destruction of the thyroid gland; therefore it is associated with other autoimmune diseases such as pernicious anaemia, vitiligo and type I diabetes mellitus.

*See Chapter 6.4, Thyroid disease.*

## 12. With regard to venous thromboembolism in pregnancy:
A. Deep venous thromboses (DVTs) usually occur in the right leg. **False**
B. Duplex ultrasound is sensitive for deep venous thromboses in the proximal leg. **True**
C. A chest X-ray should routinely be performed when investigating chest pain in the second and third trimester. **True**
D. Intravenous heparin is the first choice of treatment in the acute presentation of a deep venous thrombosis. **False**
E. Thrombolysis is contraindicated in pregnancy. **False**

The majority of DVTs occurring during pregnancy are in the left leg. An abnormal chest X-ray is found in 69–80 per cent of patients with a pulmonary embolus. Low-molecular-weight heparin by subcutaneous injection is the treatment of choice in both the pregnant and non-pregnant population. There is limited information on the use of thrombolysis in pregnancy. Streptokinase is most commonly used and does not cross the placenta; side effects include genital tract bleeding, and its use should be reserved for haemodynamically unstable patients.

*See Chapter 6.5, Haematological conditions.*

## 13. With regard to haemophilia A and B:
A. They are autosomal recessive diseases. **False**
B. Haemophilia B results from factor IX deficiency. **True**
C. Female carriers usually have normal factor VIII levels in haemophilia. **False**
D. Caesarean section is the usual mode of delivery in haemophilia pregnancies. **False**
E. Desmopressin (DDAVP) is used to increase factor IX levels. **False**

The haemophilias are X-linked conditions. As carriers have one affected gene, it is often assumed that their factor levels will be 50 per cent of normal, but levels vary markedly. There is no place for elective caesarean section, other than for obstetric indications. DDAVP can increase factor VIII levels.

*See Chapter 6.5, Haematological conditions.*

## 14. In maternal sickle cell disease:
A. The spontaneous abortion rate is increased. **True**
B. The incidence of pre-eclampsia is increased. **True**
C. The incidence of spontaneous delivery preterm is increased. **True**
D. The incidence of small-for-dates fetuses is unchanged. **False**
E. The presence of sickle cell disease in the fetus cannot be detected. **False**

In sickle cell disease, it is the structure of the globin chains that is abnormal. Pregnancies complicated by sickle cell disease are at increased risk of miscarriage, pre-eclampsia, IUGR and increased rate of caesarean sections. The disease is an autosomal recessive disorder that can be diagnosed antenatally; however, careful counselling is required as the patient may be suffering from the disease.

*See Chapter 6.5, Haematological conditions.*

### 15. The following are indicative of underlying pre-existing renal disease:

| | |
|---|---|
| A. Bilateral renal pelvi-calyceal dilatation on ultrasound. | **False** |
| B. Bilateral small kidneys on ultrasound. | **True** |
| C. Trace proteinuria and 1+ haematuria at booking at 10 weeks. | **False** |
| D. Serum creatinine of 99 μmol/L at 16 weeks in a woman weighing 59 kg. | **True** |
| E. A 24-hour urinary protein loss of 3.5 g at 12 weeks. | **True** |

Bilateral renal pelvi-calyceal dilatation is a common finding in pregnancy, whereas ultrasound appearance of bilateral small kidneys implies chronic renal failure. Urinary dipstick identifications of trace proteinuria and 1+ haematuria are both common in pregnancy, although the haematuria requires further investigation. A serum creatinine of 99 μmol/L at 16 weeks is high for a pregnant woman of this size. The upper limit of normal in the second trimester in an average-size woman is about 65 μmol/L. The upper limit of normal for 24-hour urinary protein loss throughout pregnancy is 0.3 g per 24 hours. Twelve weeks is too early for pre-eclampsia.

*See Chapter 6.6, Renal disease (and Chapter 6.2, Diabetes mellitus).*

### 16. Concerning bacteriuria in pregnancy:

| | |
|---|---|
| A. Asymptomatic bacteriuria complicates about 1 per cent of pregnancies. | **False** |
| B. Bacteriuria is considered significant if there are more than 10 000 organisms per mL of urine. | **False** |
| C. A 7-day course of antibiotics is recommended for asymptomatic bacteriuria. | **False** |
| D. A 7-day course of antibiotics is recommended for pyelonephritis. | **False** |
| E. Nitrofurantoin therapy should be avoided in the first trimester. | **False** |

The incidence of asymptomatic bacteriuria in pregnancy ranges from 4 to 7 per cent. Bacteriuria is considered significant if there are more than 100 000 organisms per mL of urine. Treatment for 3 days is sufficient for asymptomatic bacteriuria. For pyelonephritis, antibiotics should be continued for 10–14 days. Owing to a haemolytic effect, nitrofurantoin should be avoided in the third trimester.

*See Chapter 6.6, Renal disease (and Chapter 6.2, Diabetes mellitus).*

### 17. Proteinuria in pregnancy may be due to:

| | |
|---|---|
| A. The presence of systemic lupus erythematosus (SLE). | **True** |
| B. Diabetes mellitus. | **True** |
| C. Chronic glomerulonephritis. | **True** |
| D. Placental abruption without pre-eclampsia. | **True** |
| E. Essential benign hypertension. | **False** |

The most common reason for pregnancy proteinuria is chronic glomerulonephritis, and this is associated with severe IUGR. This may be an inherited condition and therefore infants should be screened postnatally. Nephropathy is a common complication of diabetes and it has the effect of doubling the risks of a poor pregnancy outcome. The presence of proteinuria in women with SLE is a strong indicator of a poor pregnancy outcome, with an increase in pre-eclampsia and IUGR.

*See Chapter 6.6, Renal disease (and Chapter 6.2, Diabetes mellitus).*

**18. The following drugs are appropriate for a woman with SLE who is 35 weeks pregnant:**

| | |
|---|---|
| A. Diclofenac. | **False** |
| B. Prednisolone. | **True** |
| C. Hydroxychloroquine. | **True** |
| D. Sulfasalazine. | **True** |
| E. Methotrexate. | **False** |

Non-steroidal anti-inflammatory drugs (NSAIDs, such as diclofenac) are often used in women with SLE. However, they are normally avoided in pregnancy because they are detrimental to the fetal kidney, causing oligohydramnios, and they may cause premature closure of the ductus arteriosus, leading to pulmonary hypertension and fetal haemorrhage in large doses. Cytotoxic drugs such as methotrexate are highly teratogenic and must be discontinued prior to pregnancy.

*See Chapter 6.7, Autoimmune conditions.*

**19. A woman with a previous stillbirth and a postpartum DVT is found to have lupus anticoagulant and medium-titre immunoglobulin M (IgM) anticardiolipin antibodies (aCL) on two occasions. In a subsequent pregnancy:**

| | |
|---|---|
| A. She has an increased risk of miscarriage. | **True** |
| B. Low-dose aspirin should be discontinued at 34 weeks. | **False** |
| C. Warfarin should be discontinued. | **True** |
| D. She does not require postpartum heparin if she has a vaginal delivery. | **False** |
| E. She requires antibiotic prophylaxis to cover delivery. | **False** |

This woman has antiphospholipid syndrome (APS). She is therefore at increased risk of early and late miscarriage, pre-eclampsia, growth restriction, abruption and premature delivery. Low-dose aspirin is the standard treatment and does not increase the risk of bleeding at the time of delivery or regional anaesthesia. There is therefore no indication to discontinue it during pregnancy. Following the diagnosis of APS, she may have been commenced on life-long warfarin or the warfarin may have been continued following her DVT. Warfarin should be discontinued once pregnancy is confirmed because it is teratogenic and increases the risk of both maternal and fetal bleeding. Heparin is used as thromboprophylaxis during pregnancy. APS is a form of acquired thrombophilia. Pregnancy, and especially the postpartum state (whatever the mode of delivery), increases the risks of thrombosis. She has had a previous DVT and therefore should receive heparin during pregnancy and postpartum. Antibiotic prophylaxis is not required for women with SLE or APS.

*See Chapter 6.7, Autoimmune conditions.*

### 20. With regard to APS:

A. It may be diagnosed if aCL or lupus anticoagulant (La) antibodies are detected in a woman who has suffered a miscarriage at less than 10 weeks.    **False**

B. It increases the risk of placental abruption.    **True**

C. Previous pregnancy outcome is the best predictor of present pregnancy outcome.    **True**

D. Fetal death is typically preceded by IUGR and oligohydramnios.    **True**

E. High-dose steroid therapy is a recommended treatment.    **False**

The diagnosis of APS can be made if either aCL or La antibodies are present in a women who has had an arterial or venous thrombosis, or has suffered three consecutive miscarriages, or one fetal death with a gestation of greater than 10 weeks' with a fetal heart present, or one premature birth secondary to pre-eclampsia or IUGR. APS significantly increases the risk of miscarriage, second and third trimester fetal death, pre-eclampsia, IUGR and placental abruption. Although high-dose steroids have been shown to improve pregnancy outcome in women with APS, steroid use is no longer justified, as the maternal side effects are too great. Low-dose aspirin has been shown to improve pregnancy outcome in this group of women. Although low-molecular-weight heparin should be given to women who have suffered a thrombosis, the benefits in women who have had no thrombosis are controversial.

*See Chapter 6.7, Autoimmune conditions.*

### 21. With regard to SLE:

A. There is in increased likelihood of an exacerbation during pregnancy.    **True**

B. There is an increased prevalence in Caucasian women.    **False**

C. The C-reactive protein (CRP) level is raised.    **False**

D. Anti-double-stranded DNA is the most common autoantibody.    **False**

E. Anti-Ro antibodies are present in 30 per cent of women with SLE.    **True**

The likelihood of a flare during pregnancy is increased by 40–60 per cent, although these episodes may be difficult to diagnose as the signs and symptoms are similar to those of pregnancy. The CRP is not raised in SLE. However, the erythrocyte sedimentation rate (ESR) is increased; this cannot be used to diagnose a flare, as pregnancy also increases the ESR. The most common autoantibody is antinuclear antibody, with the most specific being anti-double-stranded DNA.

*See Chapter 6.7, Autoimmune conditions.*

## 22. In a women with obstetric cholestasis:

A. The risk of stillbirth increases with gestation.   **True**

B. The presence of steatorrhoea increases the risk of postpartum haemorrhage.   **True**

C. The pruritus may recur with use of the combined oral contraceptive pill (COCP).   **True**

D. Recurrence in subsequent pregnancies is unlikely.   **False**

E. The treatment of choice is cholestyramine.   **False**

Most stillbirths occur at term. Steatorrhoea implies malabsorption of fat and therefore fat-soluble vitamins. This means that vitamin K deficiency and therefore postpartum haemorrhage are more likely. A genetic susceptibility to the cholestatic effect of oestrogens is thought to underlie the recurrence described with use of the COCP. Recurrence in subsequent pregnancies exceeds 90 per cent. Cholestyramine is not the treatment of choice because it is poorly tolerated, may exacerbate vitamin K deficiency and is not as successful at treating symptoms and the raised liver function tests as ursodeoxycholic acid.

*See Chapter 6.8, Liver and gastrointestinal disease.*

## 23. Intrahepatic cholestasis in pregnancy is associated with:

A. Elevation of total bile salts in the blood.   **True**

B. A positive direct Coombs' test in the neonate.   **False**

C. Elevated serum acid phosphatase activity.   **False**

D. Preterm labour.   **True**

E. Marked geographical variations.   **True**

In intrahepatic cholestasis, the serum shows an increase in conjugated bilirubin and alkaline phosphatase and not acid phosphatase. There is large geographical variation in the incidence of intrahepatic cholestasis, with one of the highest incidences occurring in Chile. The fetal risks for obstetric cholastasis include preterm labour, meconium staining and, rarely, intrauterine fetal death.

*See Chapter 6.8, Liver and gastrointestinal disease.*

## 24. Recognized causes of vomiting in the second trimester of pregnancy include:

A. Ectopic pregnancy.   **False**

B. Herpes gestationis.   **False**

C. Ulcerative colitis.   **False**

D. Acute pyelonephritis.   **True**

E. Appendicitis.   **True**

Ectopic pregnancy is associated with vomiting; however, this occurs in the first trimester not the second. Ulcerative colitis is associated with first trimester flare-ups that present as abdominal pain and diarrhoea and passage of rectal mucus and blood. Acute pyelonephritis and appendicitis are both recognized causes of vomiting in the second trimester and need to be excluded in any patient who presents with this symptom.

*See Chapter 6.8, Liver and gastrointestinal disease.*

### 25. Regarding respiratory disease in pregnancy:

A. Theophyllines are contraindicated in pregnancy. **False**

B. Pregnancy does not cause a net deterioration of cystic fibrosis. **True**

C. Congenital tuberculosis occurs in 25 per cent of cases of maternal tuberculosis (TB). **False**

D. Aciclovir should be given within 24 hours of a chickenpox rash developing. **True**

E. Women being treated for TB should be advised not to breastfeed. **False**

No commonly used anti-asthma medications are contraindicated in pregnancy, including theophyllines. Pregnancy does not appear to accelerate the gradual decline in lung function found in people with cystic fibrosis (CF), except where lung function is already very severely impaired. Vertical TB transmission in utero is extremely rare, with only a few cases on record. More common is horizontal transmission, after delivery, by infectious relatives. Women with TB are allowed to breastfeed and the commonly used drugs (isoniazid, rifampicin and ethambutol) are not a contraindication. Even in the absence of respiratory symptoms, aciclovir is recommended for women presenting early (within 24 hours) with a chickenpox rash, the aim being to limit the chances of a pneumonitis occurring.

*See Chapter 6.9, Respiratory conditions.*

### 26. With regard to tuberculosis:

A. It is caused by the organism *Mycobacterium tuberculosis*. **True**

B. Delayed treatment in pregnancy is associated with IUGR. **True**

C. Delayed treatment in pregnancy is associated with prematurity. **True**

D. Vertical transmission to the fetus is common. **False**

E. Separation of the infant from the mother is usually necessary to prevent lateral transmission. **False**

F. The drugs isoniazid, ethambutol and streptomycin are safe in pregnancy. **False**

Tuberculosis is caused by the organism *Mycobacterium tuberculosis*. The risk factors for the disease include human immunodeficiency virus (HIV)-positive status, homelessness, over-crowding and poor nutrition. The early treatment of this disease confers no risk to the fetus. However, delayed treatment has been associated with IUGR and premature delivery, as well as with an increased risk of vertical transmission. Vertical transmission to the fetus is exceptionally rare. The separation of mother and infant is not normally required, as the mother is non-infectious after 2 weeks of treatment. Streptomycin is associated with fetal eighth nerve damage, and therefore is contraindicated in pregnancy.

*See Chapter 6.9, Respiratory conditions.*

**27. A 28-year-old woman has CF and her partner is negative for the common ΔF 508 mutation. With regard to her pregnancy:**

A. The risk of their offspring being affected with CF is 1:5000.        **False**

B. Colonization with *Burkholderia cepacia* is a predictor of maternal pregnancy outcome.        **True**

C. An oral glucose tolerance test should be arranged at 26 weeks.        **True**

D. There is, on average, a 30 per cent loss of lung function with pregnancy.        **False**

E. She has only a 40 per cent chance of being alive 10 years after giving birth.        **False**

The risk of the fetus being affected by CF is 1:500. This is due to the fact that the incidence of the CF mutation is 1:25 in the population; however, 90 per cent of those will be the ΔF508. Therefore the partner has a 1:250 risk of carrier status for CF and so the fetus has a 1:500 risk of being affected. A number of different markers of disease severity have been proposed as predictors of maternal and fetal outcome; these include pre-pregnancy pulmonary function, colonization with *Burkholderia cepacia* and the presence of pulmonary hypertension. Pancreatic function is affected in women with CF, and 8 per cent will develop gestational diabetes in pregnancy. Eighty per cent of women will be alive 10 years after giving birth.

*See Chapter 6.9, Respiratory conditions.*

**28. Regarding neurological disease in pregnancy:**

A. The overall progression of multiple sclerosis (MS) is accelerated by pregnancy.        **False**

B. Women using benzodiazepines in pregnancy should receive vitamin K supplements.        **False**

C. Neonatal myasthenia occurs in no more than 50 per cent of babies born to women with myasthenia gravis.        **True**

D. The pregnancy-associated increase in stroke risk is mostly confined to the puerperium.        **True**

E. Arteriovenous malformations are a more common cause of intracerebral haemorrhage than aneurysms.        **True**

Pregnancy does not alter the overall course of MS, and there is evidence to suggest it may help to protect against its onset. However, relapses do occur more frequently than would be expected during the puerperium. Phenytoin, carbamazepine, phenobarbitone and possibly even valproate do limit vitamin K carboxylation (activation), and vitamin K supplements are advised in pregnancy. Benzodiazepines do not cause vitamin K deficiency. Neonatal myasthenia gravis occurs in 10–50 per cent of babies born to women with myasthenia gravis. The overall relative risk for stroke is between 2 and 3 during pregnancy, but this is mostly confined to the puerperium. Arteriovenous malformations (AVMs) are a less common cause of haemorrhagic stroke than aneurysms except in pregnancy. Oestrogen-induced expansion of the AVM is one possible cause for this.

*See Chapter 6.10, Neuromuscular conditions.*

## 29. Regarding MS:

A. Pregnancy affects the long-term prognosis of the disease.          **False**

B. Epidural analgesia will precipitate a relapse.          **False**

C. Attacks are more likely to occur in pregnancy.          **False**

D. Urinary urgency may be treated with tricyclic antidepressants.          **True**

E. The infant has a 10 per cent risk of developing MS later in life.          **False**

Multiple sclerosis is a relatively common (0.06–0.1 per cent) autoimmune central nervous disease, which is characterized by a relapsing and remitting course. The use of epidural analgesia has not been shown to have any effect on the course of the disease. Many patients with MS suffer from urinary symptoms and these can be safely treated with tricyclic antidepressants such as imipramine during pregnancy. The infants of mothers with MS have a 1 per cent risk of developing the disease later in life. The relapse rate is reduced during pregnancy; however, it is markedly increased in the first 3–6 months post-delivery, with approximately 40 per cent of patients suffering a relapse.

*See Chapter 6.10, Neuromuscular conditions.*

## 30. In relation to women who embark on pregnancy with a diagnosis of epilepsy:

A. Carbamazepine is associated with fetal cardiac defects.          **False**

B. Following delivery, anti-epileptic drugs may need to be reduced.          **True**

C. Vitamin K should be commenced from 30 weeks' gestation.          **False**

D. Maternal death via drowning is a recognized association of epilepsy.          **True**

E. Intravenous magnesium sulphate is the best treatment of a status epilepticus during labour.          **False**

Carbamazepine is classically associated with neural tube defects (NTDs). However, sodium valproate is associated with NTDs, genitourinary and cardiac defects, and phenytoin is associated with cardiac and genitourinary defects. Vitamin K supplementation should be commenced from 36 weeks' gestation. This is because vitamin K-dependent clotting factors within the newborn may be reduced, leading to haemorrhagic disease. The Confidential Enquiries into Maternal Deaths (CEMD) stated that 3 of the 8 deaths attributable to epilepsy were caused through drowning. It also suggests that women should be encouraged to take showers and not baths as a preventative measure. Although magnesium sulphate is the treatment of choice for an undiagnosed seizure during labour, intravenous benzodiazepines (i.e. lorazepam, diazepam) are the recognized treatment for status epilepticus during labour.

*See Chapter 6.10, Neuromuscular conditions.*

**31. Polymorphic eruption of pregnancy (PEP) is associated with:**

A. Increased rates of stillbirth.                                                    **False**

B. Approximately 1:250 pregnancies.                                          **True**

C. A typical onset in the second trimester.                                **False**

D. No fetal effects.                                                                      **True**

E. Recurrence in subsequent pregnancies.                                **False**

Pemphigoid gestationis can be confused with PEP if there are no vesicles present. Pemphigoid gestationis has been linked to increased rates of stillbirth, IUGR and preterm labour. The onset is usually in the late third trimester. Recurrence is uncommon.

*See Chapter 6.11, Dermatological conditions.*

**32. With regard to dermatological conditions in pregnancy:**

A. PEP is characterized by an abdominal rash with umbilical sparing.       **True**

B. Erythema nodosum may deteriorate or present in pregnancy.              **True**

C. Podophyllin does not cross the placenta in clinically significant amounts.    **False**

Polymorphic eruption of pregnancy is a pregnancy-specific rash with an incidence of 1:200 women. It usually presents in the third trimester with an abdominal rash. The rash characteristically has umbilical sparing. One per cent menthol in aqueous cream is the treatment of choice in this condition; however, 1% hydrocortisone may be given if necessary. Podophyllin and podophyllotoxin, which are used for the treatment of genital warts, both cross the placenta in significant amount and are teratogenic.

*See Chapter 6.11, Dermatological conditions.*

**33. Regarding substance misuse in pregnancy:**

A. Neonatal abstinence syndrome (NAS) does not occur with methadone use.       **False**

B. Cocaine acts via the central gamma-aminobutyric acid type A (GABA-A) receptor
to cause hypertension.                                                              **False**

C. A third of alcoholics produce offspring with the fetal alcohol syndrome (FAS).    **True**

D. A clear causal link exists between benzodiazepine exposure in the first trimester
and cleft lip and palate.                                                           **False**

E. Marijuana causes fetal microcephaly.                                            **False**

Methadone, like any opiate, can result in physical dependency and can therefore cause NAS. Owing to its longer half-life, the onset of the NAS after delivery may be delayed beyond that found with heroin. Cocaine causes vasoconstriction and hypertension by blocking the reuptake of catecholamines at peripheral nerve terminals. Benzodiazepines act via the GABA-A receptor and have an anxiolytic and sedative effect. Debate still exists regarding the teratogenic nature of benzodiazepines. Although the link between alcohol consumption and FAS is not a clear one either, approximately one-third of alcoholics (by definition, very heavy drinkers) will have children with FAS. Cannabis, on the other hand, has not been clearly linked with any fetal damage, although concerns do exist about potential subtle neuro-developmental effects in exposed offspring.

*See Chapter 6.12, Drug and alcohol misuse.*

### 34.  With regard to substance abuse:

A. Cannabis smoking is associated with IUGR.                                    **False**

B. Cocaethylene is a potent vasoconstrictor derived from cocaine.               **False**

C. Alcohol has abortive properties.                                             **True**

D. Cocaine is associated with macrocephaly.                                     **False**

E. Benzodiazepines in the neonate cause respiratory depression, reduced tone and
   poor feeding.                                                                **True**

Cocaethylene is a potent vasoconstrictor derived from the interaction of cocaine with alcohol.

Alcohol has been shown in animal studies to have abortifacient properties; however, this has not been shown in humans. Both cocaine and Ecstasy have been linked to neurological teratogenesis, including microcephaly.

*See Chapter 6.12, Drug and alcohol misuse.*

### 35.  Regarding methadone use in pregnancy:

A. Methadone has a shorter half-life than heroin.                               **False**

B. Naloxone should not be given to opiate-dependent mothers or their offspring. **True**

C. NAS presents within 24 hours of delivery.                                    **False**

D. Breastfeeding is contraindicated.                                            **False**

Methadone has a longer half-life than heroin. Severe withdrawal effects may occur if naloxone is given to opiate-dependent mothers or their offspring. Methadone maintenance does not prevent NAS but may delay its presentation until the second day of life due to its longer half-life. Breastfeeding is encouraged in most women, even those on methadone.

*See Chapter 6.12, Drug and alcohol misuse.*

### 36.  Smoking in pregnancy is associated with increased risks of:

A. Premature labour.                                                            **True**

B. Long-term respiratory disease amongst infants.                              **True**

C. Lowered IQs amongst offspring.                                              **True**

There are many studies that demonstrate an association between an increased risk of premature labour and smoking. Long-term effects on offspring include lowered IQs and an effect on respiratory illness over and above that which may be caused by the children living in a family where smoking continues.

*See Chapter 6.13, Smoking.*

**37. Smoking in pregnancy is associated with:**

A. An increase in the incidence of pre-eclampsia.   **False**

B. A reduction in cognitive function for the infant later in life.   **True**

C. A reduction in the infant birth weight.   **True**

D. An increase in postoperative chest infections.   **True**

E. An increase in the rate of placental abruption.   **True**

Twenty-seven per cent of women smoke during pregnancy, therefore this is a common problem. Smoking in pregnancy is associated with a 50 per cent reduction in the incidence of pre-eclampsia; however, those who do develop pre-eclampsia and smoke have worse disease when compared to those who do not smoke. Smoking is associated with an increase in both postoperative chest infection rates and thrombosis. There is an increase in the perinatal mortality rate in women who smoke, and this is partly due to an increase in the placental abruption rate. There is also an increase in the placenta praevia rate among women who smoke.

*See Chapter 6.13, Smoking.*

**38. Pregnancy is associated with increases in:**

A. Total iron-binding capacity.   **True**

B. Iron absorption.   **True**

C. Haematocrit.   **False**

D. Mean cell haemoglobin concentration (MCHC).   **False**

E. Serum ferritin concentration.   **False**

There is a moderate increase in iron absorption. The haematocrit falls, consequent upon an increase in the plasma volume, which exceeds that of the red cell mass. The MCHC remains stable. Serum iron and ferritin concentrations decrease secondary to increased utilization.

*See Chapter 7.1, Anaemia.*

**39. In pregnancy:**

A. A haemoglobin concentration of 11 g/dL is the lower limit of normal according
   to the World Health Organization (WHO).   **True**

B. A low serum iron with a low total iron-binding capacity suggests iron deficiency.   **False**

C. The overall total iron requirement is approximately 1 g.   **True**

D. Iron absorption from the jejunum is increased.   **True**

E. Iron should be advised for all pregnant women.   **False**

In practice, 10 g/dL may be a better cut-off. A high total iron binding capacity and low serum ferritin diagnoses iron deficiency anaemia. There is no evidence that iron is of benefit to all pregnant women, as the only proven benefit is to increase iron stores. It is therefore more appropriate to search for anaemia rather than to treat all women with iron, as some may experience side effects.

*See Chapter 7.1, Anaemia.*

### 40. With regard to acute appendicitis in pregnancy:

A. It is more common than outside pregnancy.                                    **False**

B. It is associated with preterm rupture of membranes.                          **True**

C. Caesarean section should not be performed at the same time as an
   appendicectomy.                                                              **True**

D. Maternal mortality exceeds 5 per cent.                                       **False**

Acute appendicitis complicates between 1:1500 and 1:2500 pregnancies; the incidence approximates to that outside pregnancy. Caesarean section should not be performed at the same time as the appendicectomy, even if the fetus is mature, because of the danger of endometritis and a significantly higher morbidity. The mortality from appendicitis in pregnancy varies; although figures as high as 2 per cent have been reported, more recent series quote lower figures.

*See Chapter 7.2, Abdominal pain.*

### 41. With regard to abdominal pain in the third trimester of pregnancy:

A. An ultrasound scan can exclude a placental abruption.                        **False**

B. Appendicitis is characterized by maximum tenderness over McBurney's point.   **False**

C. Round ligament pain is the most common cause.                               **False**

D. Acute pyelonephritis is more likely on the left than on the right.          **False**

Placental abruption is more likely to occur in the second and third trimesters. The diagnosis may be difficult in cases where there is no overt vaginal bleeding. Although an ultrasound scan may be useful in establishing the diagnosis, it cannot exclude the diagnosis, as approximately a 500 mL retroplacental haemorrhage is required before an abruption can reliably be visualized. The incidence of appendicitis in pregnancy is approximately the same as in the non-pregnant population. However, due to the displacement of the bowel by the uterus, the maximal tenderness in the third trimester occurs in the flank. Round ligament pain occurs in up to 30 per cent of pregnant women; however, it most commonly occurs in the late first and early second trimesters. Acute pyelonephritis is the most common cause of renal pain; dextro-rotation of the uterus increases the risk of it occurring on the right-hand side.

*See Chapter 7.2, Abdominal pain.*

## 42.  Regarding cancer arising during pregnancy:

A. Chemotherapy must never be given during the first trimester.                                **False**

B. The long-term survival after diagnosis of melanoma is adversely affected by
pregnancy.                                                                                     **False**

C. The maximum recommended radiation exposure during pregnancy is 5 Gray.        **False**

D. Treatment of cervical intraepithelial neoplasia (CIN) is usually delayed until after
delivery.                                                                                      **True**

E. Breast cancer is the most common cancer to be diagnosed during pregnancy.      **False**

Although the risk of fetal harm is much greater in the first trimester, numerous reports exist
of normal outcomes following chemotherapy use during the first 12 weeks of pregnancy. In-
depth counselling is needed to explore management options. Whereas some couples will
choose to have a termination, others will accept the risk to their baby and go ahead with
chemotherapy whilst continuing the pregnancy. Some will even choose to delay maternal
therapy until the fetal risk is more acceptable. Case-controlled studies show that pregnancy
does not affect the prognosis for survival after melanoma, even if this is diagnosed during
pregnancy. A dose of 5 rad (0.05 Gy) is considered a safe level of radiation exposure during
pregnancy, although reports exist suggesting possible harm with levels as low as 1–2 rad.

Cervical intraepithelial neoplasia should be observed closely during pregnancy using
colposcopy and directed biopsies (if there is any suggestion of invasion). Treatments for CIN,
such as large loop excision of the transformation zone (LLETZ) and knife cone biopsy, should
be reserved for the puerperium unless invasion is confirmed by directed biopsy, as they are
associated with a significantly greater chance of haemorrhage. Cervical cancer is more
commonly diagnosed during pregnancy (1 in 1200) than breast cancer (1 in 3000).

*See Chapter 7.3, Malignancy.*

## 43. With regard to cancer in pregnancy:

| | |
|---|---|
| A. Twenty-five per cent of cancers presenting in pregnancy are breast cancers. | **True** |
| B. Technetium bone scans are indicated. | **True** |
| C. Radical hysterectomy is mandatory for micro-invasive cervical cancer. | **False** |
| D. Cervical cancer is an indication for a classical caesarean section. | **True** |
| E. Hodgkin's lymphoma must be treated immediately upon diagnosis. | **False** |

Cervical cancer in the form of an abnormal smear is the commonest cancer to present during pregnancy. However, breast cancer constitutes 25 per cent of all cancers in pregnancy, with an incidence of 1:3000. Technetium bone scans can be used if necessary, as the total dose is less than 0.5 rad. Frank invasive cancer of the cervix is uncommon in pregnancy; however, abnormal smears are the most common reason for gynaecological oncological referral. Macro-invasive disease can be managed as in the non-pregnant women, with initially a knife cone biopsy. Higher-grade lesions (Stage Ib–IIa) require radical hysterectomy and, if the gestation is greater than 20 weeks, delaying delivery until fetal maturity is achieved should be discussed. Delivery in these cases should be by classical caesarean section to avoid trauma to the lower genital tract. The treatment for Hodgkin's lymphoma and chronic myeloid leukaemia can often be delayed until after the pregnancy. Acute leukaemias and non-Hodgkin's lymphoma must be treated immediately, as the risks to the woman and her pregnancy from haemorrhage, anaemia and sepsis outweigh any possible fetal effects from therapy.

*See Chapter 7.3, Malignancy.*

## 44. With regard to HIV in pregnancy:

| | |
|---|---|
| A. A positive HIV blood test in pregnancy is not reliable. | **False** |
| B. A low maternal CD4 count increases the mother-to-child transmission of HIV. | **True** |
| C. A high maternal HIV RNA load increases the mother-to-child transmission of HIV. | **True** |
| D. Use of antiretroviral agents is always commenced in the first trimester of pregnancy. | **False** |
| E. HIV infection increases the mother-to-child transmission of the hepatitis C virus. | **True** |
| F. If there are ruptured membranes for 6 hours, there is no advantage to delivery by caesarean section. | **False** |

A positive HIV blood test is as dependable in pregnancy as it is outside pregnancy – and is a reliable guide to infection. Therapy should be individualized and based on the woman's clinical, virological and immunological status, as well as the gestational age of the fetus. For women diagnosed with HIV infection during the first trimester, treatment should be delayed until the second trimester. There is an increase in the vertical transmission once the membranes have been ruptured for 4 hours. However, if a woman presents with this history, delivery by caesarean section is still recommended.

*See Chapter 7.4, Infection.*

### 45. With regard to viral infection in pregnancy:

A. The majority of genital herpes is caused by type 2 herpes simplex virus (HSV).    **True**

B. Initial treatment for HSV in pregnancy should include a penicillin.    **False**

C. Shingles in pregnancy does not appear to cause fetal sequelae.    **True**

D. Cytomegalovirus (CMV) is associated with non-immune fetal hydrops.    **True**

Initial genital or oral HSV infection can be treated with topical, oral or intravenous aciclovir; secondary infection is treated with antibiotics.

*See Chapter 7.4, Infection.*

### 46. Chlamydial infection in pregnancy:

A. Has an incubation period of up to 21 days.    **True**

B. Is typically asymptomatic.    **True**

C. Can present with perihepatitis.    **True**

D. Should be treated with tetracycline.    **False**

E. Can cause postpartum endometritis.    **True**

The incubation period is 7–21 days. A perihepatitis can occur – the Fitz–Hugh–Curtis syndrome. Tetracyclines are contraindicated in pregnancy; acceptable alternatives are amoxycillin or erythromycin.

*See Chapter 7.4, Infection.*

### 47. Congenital infection with CMV:

A. Is associated with hepatosplenomegaly.    **True**

B. Is associated with intracerebral calcification.    **True**

C. Is a cause of microcephaly.    **True**

D. Will result in symptoms in 5–10 per cent of babies at birth.    **True**

E. Is a cause of polyhydramnios.    **True**

Congenital CMV is associated with various fetal manifestations. These include hepato-splenomegaly, microcephaly, IUGR, hyperbilirubinaemia, intracerebral calcification and mental retardation. Only 5–10 per cent of infants are symptomatic at birth. Congenital CMV is a cause of fetal hydrops and thus polyhydramnios.

*See Chapter 7.4, Infection.*

### 48. *Listeria monocytogenes*:

A. Is a Gram-negative anaerobe.    **False**

B. Is carried in the intestinal tract of 20 per cent of the population.    **False**

C. Is spread through droplets in the air.    **False**

D. Is a spore-forming bacterium.    **False**

E. Is associated with meconium staining of the liquor amnii in premature gestations.    **True**

*Listeria monocytogenes* is a Gram-positive, beta-haemolytic anaerobic bacterium. It is carried in 5–10 per cent of the adult population of the UK. It is spread through raw foods and soft cheeses, which are best avoided during pregnancy. *Listeria monocytogenes* is not spore forming; however, it is resistant to the effects of freezing and heat.

*See Chapter 7.4, Infection.*

## 49. Gestational diabetes diagnosed for the first time during pregnancy is characteristically associated with:

| | |
|---|---|
| A. An increased risk of developing diabetes mellitus later in life. | **True** |
| B. A need for treatment with insulin in the majority of cases. | **False** |
| C. An increased incidence of fetal malformations, even when treated. | **False** |
| D. A decreased risk of pre-eclampsia. | **False** |
| E. An increased risk of fetal respiratory distress syndrome. | **True** |

Gestational diabetes is defined as carbohydrate intolerance that begins or is first recognized during pregnancy and, in most cases, resolves after pregnancy. Women who are diagnosed as having gestational diabetes in pregnancy have a 40–60 per cent increased risk of developing non-insulin-dependent diabetes within the following 20 years. Gestational diabetes confers several risks to both the mother and the fetus. Maternal risks include pre-eclampsia, pregnancy-induced hypertension and increased risk of operative deliveries. Fetal risks include macrosomia, preterm delivery, unexplained stillbirth and respiratory distress.

*See Chapter 7.5, Gestational diabetes.*

## 50. Screening tests for diabetes in pregnancy include:

| | |
|---|---|
| A. Performing glycosylated haemoglobin estimations on all women who have had a macrosomic baby (>4.5 kg). | **False** |
| B. Random blood sampling at 28–32 weeks. | **True** |
| C. A 50 g glucose load at booking. | **True** |
| D. A 50 g glucose load at 28 weeks if potential diabetic features pertain. | **True** |
| E. Glucose testing of the urine. | **True** |

Many studies have investigated the use of glycosylated haemoglobin and it has been shown to have a poor sensitivity. Testing for glycosuria at each antenatal visit remains a cheap, simple and established method of screening. The sensitivity of this test is low, but the specificity is high; about 90 per cent of the pregnant population do not have random glycosuria. The low sensitivity means that a further test is required.

*See Chapter 7.5, Gestational diabetes.*

### 51. The incidence of pre-eclampsia is:

A. Increased in teenage pregnancies. **True**

B. Increased in pregnancies complicated by hydrops fetalis. **True**

C. Doubled by a family history in a first-degree relative. **False**

D. Increased in women with gestational diabetes. **True**

E. Approximately 20 per cent if there is notching on uterine artery Doppler waveform analysis at 20 weeks. **True**

F. Reduced by prophylactic fish oil administration. **False**

Risk may be related to the size of the placenta; molar pregnancies have been associated with pre-eclampsia, as have pregnancies complicated by hydrops fetalis (mirror syndrome). A family history in a first-degree relative increases the risk of pre-eclampsia four–eight-fold. All forms of glucose intolerance, including gestational diabetes, are associated with an increased risk; this may be related to obesity. At 20 weeks' gestation in a low-risk population, approximately 1 in 5 women will develop pre-eclampsia if they have an abnormal waveform. Four trials of fish oil administration have not shown any reduction in the incidence of pre-eclampsia.

*See Chapter 7.6, Pre-eclampsia and non-proteinuric pregnancy-induced hypertension.*

### 52. With regard to eclampsia:

A. Eighteen per cent of eclamptic seizures occur in the postnatal period. **False**

B. Magnesium sulphate administration is associated with fetal hypercalcaemia. **False**

C. Magnesium sulphate can only be given intravenously. **False**

D. The commonest cause of maternal death is cerebral vascular accident. **False**

E. It is a recognized cause of cortical blindness. **True**

The greater proportion of eclamptic seizures occurs in the postnatal period (44 per cent); 38 per cent occur antenatally and 18 per cent during labour. Magnesium sulphate administration is associated with neonatal hypotonia, hypocalcaemia and respiratory depression. It may also be given intramuscularly if no intravenous access can be established. Maternal complications of magnesium sulphate administration include headaches, palpitations, paralytic ileus, pulmonary oedema and respiratory depression. The commonest cause of maternal death from eclampsia is adult respiratory distress syndrome.

*See Chapter 7.6, Pre-eclampsia and non-proteinuric pregnancy-induced hypertension.*

### 53. In HELLP (haemolysis, increased liver enzymes and low platelets) syndrome:

A. Most patients are in the immediate postpartum state.                          **False**

B. Platelet count falls below $100 \times 10^9/L$.                                **True**

C. The recurrence rate is 40–60 per cent if the index pregnancy diagnosis was after
32 weeks.                                                                        **False**

D. The lactate dehydrogenase concentration falls.                                **False**

E. Profound vasodilatation occurs.                                               **False**

The recurrence rate for HELLP syndrome is dependent on the gestation at diagnosis of the index pregnancy. The recurrence rate has been reported as between 40 and 60 per cent if the initial presentation was less than 32 weeks; however, this is reduced to 15 per cent if the diagnosis was made after 32 weeks of gestation. In HELLP syndrome the lactate dehydrogenase concentration is elevated due to renal involvement. HELLP syndrome is a severe variant of pre-eclampsia and therefore there is profound vasoconstriction not dilatation.

*See Chapter 7.6, Pre-eclampsia and non-proteinuric pregnancy-induced hypertension.*

### 54. Concerning the administration of drugs in pregnancy:

A. Highly lipid-soluble drugs administered via the respiratory system reach higher
concentrations in the plasma at a faster rate in pregnant than in non-pregnant
women.                                                                           **True**

B. Anti-metabolites administered in pregnancy are associated with preterm labour.   **False**

C. Carbamazepine is the safest anticonvulsant agent in pregnancy.                **False**

D. When administered in the third trimester, beta-blockers may cause fetal
hyperglycaemia.                                                                  **True**

E. When cholera vaccines are administered in the first trimester, termination of
pregnancy should be offered.                                                     **False**

F. Acetaminophen (paracetamol) is considered the analgesic of choice in pregnancy.   **True**

Anti-metabolites interfere with cell division and are therefore associated with a spectrum of malformations. Most of the anti-epileptic drugs, including carbamazepine, are teratogenic. Carbamazepine is associated with a pattern of malformations similar to those induced by the hydantoin group. In addition, carbamazepine induces NTDs. If indicated, killed vaccines such as those for cholera can be given to pregnant women without risk to the fetus.

*See Chapter 8, Medication in pregnancy.*

### 55. The following are teratogenic consequences of drug administration in pregnancy:

A. Tetracycline: yellowish coloration of the teeth.    **False**

B. Phenytoin: cleft lip and palate.    **True**

C. Sodium valproate: NTDs.    **True**

D. Heparin: nasal hypoplasia.    **False**

E. Zidovudine (AZT): skull defects.    **False**

F. Penicillin: cardiac defects    **False**

Yellowish coloration of the teeth is a non-teratogenic consequence of tetracycline administration. Approximately one-third of children born to mothers on phenytoin have minor anomalies and 10 per cent have major anomalies. Heparin is a large-molecular-weight molecule and does not cross the placenta; the teratogenic effects of warfarin include nasal hypoplasia. AZT is generally regarded as safe. Penicillin and its derivatives are not teratogenic.

*See Chapter 8, Medication in pregnancy.*

### 56. Concerning the use of antibiotics in pregnancy:

A. Erythromycin does not cross the placenta.    **True**

B. Trimethoprim is associated with the neonatal grey baby syndrome.    **False**

C. Streptomycin is associated with sensorineural deafness.    **True**

D. Erythromycin is the drug of choice in patients with premature rupture of fetal membranes.    **True**

E. Cephalosporins are associated with neonatal jaundice.    **False**

Chloramphenicol is associated with the neonatal grey baby syndrome. Sulphonamides cross the placenta and may compete with the binding of bilirubin in the fetus, resulting in neonatal jaundice.

*See Chapter 8, Medication in pregnancy.*

### 57. The following drugs are correctly paired with the following complications:

A. Carbimazole: fetal goitre.    **True**

B. Warfarin: fetal chondrodysplasia.    **True**

C. Labetalol: IUGR.    **True**

D. Sodium valproate: NTDs.    **True**

E. Lithium: cardiac malformations.    **True**

Carbimazole is used in the treatment of maternal hyperthyroidism. It crosses the placenta and has been shown to cause fetal hypothyroidism, which leads to a fetal goitre developing. Maternal treatment with warfarin is associated with fetal warfarin syndrome, which is characterized by microcephaly, nasal hypoplasia, stippled bone epiphyses, hydrocephaly and chondrodysplasia. The anti-hypertensive labetolol has been associated with IUGR and fetal bradycardias. Sodium valproate is associated with NTDs and genitourinary and cardiac defects.

*See Chapter 8, Medication in pregnancy.*

### 58. With regard to maternal mortalities:

A. They include those deaths caused by ectopic pregnancies.  **True**

B. Forty per cent of the maternal deaths in the UK occur in social class 1.  **False**

C. Their incidence is higher in patients over the age of 40.  **True**

D. Epilepsy is the commonest cause of indirect maternal death.  **False**

E. In the UK, Asian women have a reduced likelihood of death in pregnancy (in comparison to Caucasian women).  **False**

Maternal death is defined as the death of a woman while pregnant or within 42 days of termination of pregnancy, from any cause related to or aggravated by the pregnancy or its management, but not from accidental or incidental causes. Low social class has a strong association with maternal death, 40 per cent of total maternal deaths occurring in social class 9. The commonest indirect cause of maternal death is cardiac disease; suicide is the next most common cause. In the last Confidential Enquiry, Asian women were three times more likely to die during pregnancy than Caucasian women.

*See Chapter 9, Maternal mortality.*

### 59. From data for the UK from the 2001 Confidential Enquiry into Stillbirths and Deaths in Infancy (CESDI):

A. Congenital anomalies are responsible for 1 in 5 pregnancy losses.  **False**

B. Abruptio placentae is associated with 50 per cent of stillbirths.  **False**

C. Intrapartum asphyxia is responsible for 20 per cent of fetal deaths.  **False**

D. The largest percentage is 'unexplained'.  **True**

From these data (CESDI, 2001) for stillbirths according to the extended Wigglesworth classification, the largest proportion of deaths was unexplained antepartum death (70 per cent); as many as 40 per cent of these may exhibit findings of IUGR. The most common identifiable causes are congenital malformations (12.2 per cent) and intrapartum-related events (9.2 per cent). Antepartum haemorrhage is associated with 15.7 per cent of all stillbirths.

*See Chapter 11, Previous history of fetal loss.*

### 60. With regard to APS:

A. It may be associated with unexplained stillbirth.  **True**

B. A single positive aCL titre is diagnostic of this condition.  **False**

C. Association with pulmonary hypertension is of little consequence.  **False**

D. Aspirin alone is the pharmacotherapy of choice.  **False**

Antiphospholipid syndrome is a prothrombotic syndrome associated with an increased risk of perinatal mortality and loss in each trimester. It can be associated with thrombosis in the placenta or extraplacental, the most significant being pulmonary embolism. Multiple pulmonary embolism may be associated with pulmonary hypertension, which carries a maternal mortality of 60 per cent. Optimal pharmacotherapy is low-dose aspirin and low-molecular-weight heparin, but for an intrauterine death after 24 weeks of gestation, no study has demonstrated improved outcome (in variance to studies for recurrent miscarriage).

*See Chapter 11, Previous history of fetal loss.*

### 61. In monochorionic pregnancies:

A. There are intraplacental vascular anastomoses.                                   **True**

B. Perinatal mortality is increased after 28 weeks.                                 **True**

C. A discordancy in first trimester nuchal translucency (NT) could denote different risks of aneuploidy.                                                               **False**

D. There is a lower risk of twin–twin transfusion syndrome (TTTS) than in dichorionic twinning.                                                                         **False**

E. Twins are always monozygous.                                                     **False**

Monochorionic twins are formed when splitting of the early cell mass occurs after 3 post-fertilization days (3–8 in monochorionic/diamniotic and 8–10 days in monochorionic/monoamniotic). On ultrasound examination, a single placental disc is visualized from the first trimester and histologically this contains deep and superficial vascular anastomoses. Most, but not all, monochorionic twins are monozygotic. However, it is possible for the fetuses to have a different genomic mix and thus karyotype. Statistically, discordant NT is associated with a 45 per cent risk of TTTS. Perinatal mortality is increased in monochorionic twinning, as compared to dichoronic twins, mostly because of the risks of TTTS.

*See Chapter 12, Multiple pregnancy.*

### 62. In TTTS:

A. The smaller twin is the recipient.                                               **False**

B. The smaller twin has the greatest risk of cardiac compromise.                    **False**

C. The larger twin is often 'stuck' to the uterine wall.                            **False**

D. Serial amnioreduction improves perinatal survival.                               **True**

E. Fetoscopic laser ablation of the placental vessels increases survival for both twins.                                                                              **False**

Twin–twin transfusion syndrome is a morbid condition affecting 1 in 5 of monochorionic twin pregnancies. The aetiology is largely unknown, but it is associated with intraplacental vascular anastomosis. As this disease progresses, the small twin (the donor) has associated oligohydramnios and becomes 'stuck' to the uterine wall. This fetus often demonstrates signs of fetal hypoperfusion, with a small bladder and aberrant umbilical artery Doppler velocimetry. The larger twin (recipient) is relatively hyperperfused, with an easily visualized fetal bladder and surrounded by excess liquor. This twin is often compromised by high-output cardiac failure and potentially hydrops. Serial amnioreduction, septostomy and fetoscopic laser ablation of placental vessels all improve prognosis and survival overall to approximately 65 per cent. There are some data indicating that fetoscopic laser ablation of placental vessels improves the survival in only one twin and is associated with significantly less infant morbidity, especially cerebral palsy.

*See Chapter 12, Multiple pregnancy.*

## 63. In ultrasound screening for chorionicity:

A. The sensitivity and specificity of defining chorionicity are improved after 16 weeks of gestation. **False**

B. A 'twin peak' or 'lambda sign' is associated with dichorionicity. **True**

C. A thick dividing amniotic membrane is present in monochorionicity. **False**

D. Same fetal sex excludes dichorionicity. **False**

E. A single placental mass is indicative of monochorionicity in the first trimester. **True**

Twenty per cent of twins are monochorionic and such pregnancies are associated with almost a 26 per cent risk of perinatal mortality. Dizygous twins can only be dichorionic diamniotic, whereas monozygous twins may be dichorionic diamniotic, monochorionic diamniotic or monochorionic monoamniotic, depending on the timing of embryo splitting.

In the first trimester, chorionicity may be determined with almost 100 per cent accuracy. In contrast, mid-trimester assessment is only 80–90 per cent accurate. If two placentae are visualized or if the fetuses are discordant for gender, the pregnancy must be dichorionic. Visualization of the **twin-peak** or **lambda** sign is also useful in the diagnosis of dichorionicity; however, the absence of this sign is not as reliable in the confirmation of monochorionicity. The identification of an arterial–arterial anastomosis by colour Doppler insonation of the chorionic plate confirms monochorionicity. Membrane thickness has also been used to assign chorionicity. In difficult cases, zygosity studies may need to be performed.

*See Chapter 12, Multiple pregnancy.*

## 64. With regard to CMV:

A. It is an RNA virus. **False**

B. It causes primary infection in 25–40 per cent of cases. **False**

C. It may cause fetal IUGR. **True**

D. Ganciclovir administered to the fetus has proven efficacy – demonstrated in randomized, controlled trials (RCTs). **False**

E. It is associated with cerebral calcification. **True**

Cytomegalovirus is a DNA, herpes-type virus. In the UK, between 50 and 85 per cent of pregnant women are immune at booking. Of the susceptible subjects, 1–4 per cent have a primary infection.

In-utero infection may cause IUGR, microcephaly, thrombocytopenia, hepatosplenomegaly and cerebral calcification.

Although fetal administration of ganciclovir has been described anecdotally, its use is not proven in RCTs.

*See Chapter 13, Fetal infections.*

### 65.  Human parvovirus B19:

A. Is a DNA virus.                                                    **True**
B. Is transmitted as a respiratory infection of children.            **True**
C. Has an incubation period of up to 6 weeks.                        **False**
D. Has predilection to fetal erythrocyte progenitor cells.           **True**
E. Crosses the placenta in <10 per cent of cases.                    **False**

Human parvovirus B19 is a small DNA virus that causes the respiratory virus illness Fifth's disease in children. It has an incubation period of up to 20 days. Approximately 50 per cent of pregnant women are not immune to human parvovirus B19. It has a transplacental passage rate of 1 in 3 and may cause significant fetal anaemia by suppressing erythrocyte progenitor cell production. It is a self-limiting infection and, if the fetal anaemia is treated, the long-term outlook is excellent.

*See Chapter 13, Fetal infections.*

### 66.  With regard to antenatal cardiotocography (CTG):

A. One acceleration of heart rate 15 beats per minute (bpm) above the baseline
   lasting 15 seconds is reassuring.                                 **False**
B. Vibroacoustic stimulation reduces the number of unreactive traces.   **True**
C. It is more predictive of fetal death than absent end-diastolic umbilical artery
   Doppler velocimetry.                                              **False**
D. It has a strong effect on improved perinatal mortality.           **False**

A normal CTG would be considered to have at least two accelerations of heart rate 15 bpm above the baseline lasting 15 seconds. Antenatal CTG has not been demonstrated to improve perinatal mortality (as assessed in 13 trials and four RCTs). Umbilical Doppler velocimetry appears to be a better predictor of perinatal outcome.

*See Chapter 14, Tests of fetal well-being.*

### 67. The ultrasound biophysical profile (BPP):

| | |
|---|---|
| A. Has a low false-negative rate. | **True** |
| B. Has a predictive negative value of 35 per cent for perinatal mortality. | **False** |
| C. Includes liquor volume assessment as part of the test. | **True** |
| D. Has proven value in preventing perinatal mortality in RCTs. | **False** |

Assessment of fetal activity has been used as a predictor of fetal compromise, with perhaps the best known system being described by Manning et al. in 1980. This BPP depends on the ultrasonic assessment over 30 minutes of liquor, fetal tone, body and breathing movements, and finally antenatal CTG. Each component is scored as normal (2) or abnormal (0), with a maximum of 10 and scores under 8 being regarded as abnormal. Observational data based on more than 80 000 high-risk pregnancies show that BPP has a negative predictive value of 99.95 per cent and a positive predictive value of 35 per cent for perinatal morbidity, including low Apgar scores, acidaemia at birth, fetal distress and fetal growth restriction. It must be remembered, however, that adverse outcomes are rare, and therefore the false-negative rates of BPP will inevitably be low. In addition, although there does appear to be a direct relationship between an abnormal BPP and adverse perinatal outcomes, even a borderline score (6) is associated with a six-fold increase in perinatal mortality rates, indicating that the test may not give sufficient warning to allow effective intervention.

The BPP is a difficult and time-consuming test to perform; cessation of movements can occur for up to 40–60 minutes due to cycling in fetal behavioural states. Systematic review of four RCTs has failed to demonstrate any significant benefit of BPP on pregnancy outcome when compared to conventional assessment.

*See Chapter 14, Tests of fetal well-being.*

### 68. Ultrasound parameters indicative of fetal growth restriction include:

| | |
|---|---|
| A. Oligohydramnios. | **True** |
| B. A symphysis–fundal height <3rd centile. | **False** |
| C. An abdominal circumference (AC) <10th centile. | **True** |
| D. Aberrant middle cerebral artery to umbilical artery Doppler pulsatility index (PI) ratio. | **True** |
| E. A change in growth velocity ($\delta$AC <1 standard deviation (SD) in 14 days). | **True** |

The ultrasound diagnosis of IUGR includes three of the following:

    oligohydramnios

    AC <10th centile for gestation

    a change in $\delta$AC <1 SD in 14 days

    aberrant middle cerebral artery:umbilical artery Doppler PI ratio.

*See Chapter 15, Fetal growth restriction.*

## 69. With regard to fetal growth restriction:

A. The perinatal mortality is lower for gestational age than for appropriately grown babies.                                                                                     **False**
B. There is a decreased risk of pulmonary haemorrhage in neonatal life.              **False**
C. It may be associated with elevated maternal serum alpha-fetoprotein (aFP) and beta-human chorionic gonadotrophin (βhCG).                                     **True**
D. It is more sensitively detected using customized growth charts.                   **True**

In IUGR, the perinatal mortality is higher than for an appropriately grown baby, and the risk of pulmonary haemorrhage is increased. Thus survival data should be based upon both gestational age and estimated weight. There is an association between elevated maternal serum aFP and βhCG and IUGR. This is partially due to the association with chromosomal anomalies, such as triploidy, but also to an association with placental insufficiency.

*See Chapter 15, Fetal growth restriction.*

## 70. Oligohydramnios:

A. Is commonly associated with amniorrhexis.                                          **True**
B. Is associated at 16 weeks with a >90 per cent risk of pulmonary hypoplasia.       **True**
C. May cause postural anomalies in the fetus.                                        **True**
D. Is commonly found in diabetic pregnancies.                                        **False**

Pre-labour, ruptured membranes or amniorrhexis are a common cause of oligohydramnios. The association with pulmonary hypoplasia is stronger the earlier it is noted in gestation. Between 16 and 20 weeks, there is at least a 90 per cent association with pulmonary hypoplasia. However, ultrasound is unable to predict which cases will be affected. Prolonged oligohydramnios will lead to postural anomalies (i.e. talipes). Diabetic pregnancies are often associated with polyhydramnios.

*See Chapter 16, Abberant liquor volume.*

## 71. With regard to polyhydramnios:

A. Increased amniotic fluid index has a detrimental effect on uterine blood flow.    **True**
B. It may be associated with fetal oesophageal atresia.                              **True**
C. It is commonly associated with the 'donor' twin in TTTS.                          **False**
D. It may be safely managed with indomethacin in the third trimester.                **False**
E. It is diagnosed in 3 per cent of all pregnancies.                                 **True**

Polyhydramnios is defined as an amniotic fluid index of >95% confidence interval (CI) for gestation and occurs in 3 per cent of all pregnancies. It can occur in any syndrome of fetal bowel obstruction or impairment of swallowing, including oesophageal atresia. It may be noted in the 'recipient' twin of TTTS. Indomethacin is best avoided in the third trimester of pregnancy, because of the risk of premature ductal closure in utero.

*See Chapter 16, Abberant liquor volume.*

### 72. Fetal hydrops is commonly caused by:

A. Anti-Duffy antibodies.                            **False**
B. Maternal human parvovirus B19 infection.          **True**
C. Fetal tachydysrhythmias.                          **True**
D. Fetal akinesia syndromes.                         **True**

Fetal hydrops is defined as fluid in two or more body cavities in the presence of skin oedema. The diagnosis is commonly made on ultrasound. Maternal alloimmunization, commonly secondary to anti-D, c and Kell antibodies, may cause severe fetal anaemia and hydrops fetalis. Human parvovirus may cause severe fetal anaemia. Conditions in which there is limited movement may cause hydrops. Cardiac failure, especially secondary to diastolic filling anomalies (as in supraventricular tachycardia), may be associated with hydrops fetalis.
*See Chapter 17, Fetal hydrops.*

### 73. Fetal hydrops can be caused by:

A. Increased fetal hydrostatic pressure.             **True**
B. Reduced oncotic pressure.                         **True**
C. Fetal tumours.                                    **True**
D. Fetal polycythaemia.                              **False**

Starling's law of fluid distribution explains the aetiology of hydrops. An increase in arterial or venous hydrostatic pressure, a reduction in oncotic pressure (i.e. hypoalbuminaemia) or increased capillary leakiness may cause increased interstitial fluid accumulation. Fetal tumours, such as sacro-coccygeal teratomas, may cause high-output cardiac failure, as may severe fetal anaemia.
*See Chapter 17, Fetal hydrops.*

### 74. For term breech presentations:

A. The incidence is 3–4 per cent.                    **True**
B. Planned caesarean delivery reduces perinatal morbidity by 75 per cent.   **True**
C. Caesarean section has been shown to reduce perinatal morbidity in those presenting in labour.   **False**
D. All women should be offered external cephalic version (ECV).   **True**

The incidence of breech presentation at term is 3–4 per cent (compared to 20 per cent at 28 weeks). If noted at term, it is a Royal College of Obstetricians and Gynaecologists (RCOG) recommendation that all women be offered ECV. The Term Breech Trial noted a significant reduction in prenatal mortality in the elective caesarean group (odds ratio (OR) 0.23, 95% CI 0.07–0.8). However, it did not examine the effects on perinatal mortality when a women presents in labour with a term breech.
*See Chapter 18, Malpresentation.*

## 75. With regard to ECV for term breech presentation:

| | |
|---|---|
| A. Fetal heart activity should be documented. | **True** |
| B. Tocolysis is always required. | **False** |
| C. It is less likely to be successful in a multiparous woman. | **False** |
| D. It reduces the need for caesarean section. | **True** |
| E. Anti-D should be administered to Rhesus-negative women. | **True** |

External cephalic version has been demonstrated to reduce the likelihood of a caesarean section significantly in pregnancies where there is a term breech presentation (OR 0.4, 95% CI 0.3–0.6), and should be offered between 37 and 42 weeks. Tocolysis is effective but does not have to be used if the uterus is relaxed. In the UK, the ECV success rate is 46 per cent. The likelihood of success increases in association with:

multiparity

adequate liquor volume

non-engagement of the presenting part.

*See Chapter 18, Malpresentation.*

## 76. Prolonged pregnancy:

| | |
|---|---|
| A. Occurs in between 8 and 14 per cent of pregnancies. | **True** |
| B. Is associated with an increased risk of stillbirth after 43 weeks. | **True** |
| C. Is associated with an increase risk of maternal haemorrhage. | **True** |
| D. Should be managed by induction of labour at 41+ weeks. | **True** |
| E. Incidence is reduced with early ultrasound dating. | **True** |

Systematic reviews and meta-analyses indicate that early ultrasound scanning reduces the incidence of prolonged pregnancy. Scandinavian series indicate that the prevalence of prolonged pregnancy (>42 weeks) is between 8 and 14 per cent. Systematic reviews indicate that induction of labour after 41+ weeks reduces perinatal mortality.

*See Chapter 19, Prolonged pregnancy.*

## 77. The following interventions are supported by high-grade evidence to reduce surgical intervention in low-risk labour:

| | |
|---|---|
| A. Preparation and support of the woman in labour. | **True** |
| B. Routine amniotomy. | **False** |
| C. Epidural analgesia. | **False** |
| D. Presence of 'Doula' support. | **True** |
| E. Continuous electronic fetal heart rate monitoring. | **False** |

Randomized, controlled trials and meta-analysis have shown that routine amniotomy shortens labour but does not improve clinical outcome. Continuous electronic fetal monitoring in low-risk labour increases operative intervention without strong evidence for improved neonatal outcome. Epidurals slow progress in labour but probably do not increase surgical intervention as one trial showed – there is, however, no improvement. Preparation and support of the woman in labour and use of Doulas do reduce the need for analgesia and decrease operative delivery.

*See Chapter 20, Routine intrapartum care: an overview.*

## 78. Cervicography gives:

A. Reliable information in the latent phase.                                              **False**

B. Reliable information in the active phase.                                              **True**

C. Prospective identification of aberrant progress.                                      **True**

D. Diagnosis of underlying pathology when there is poor progress.                        **False**

E. Good predictive value for operative delivery (2-hour action line).                    **False**

Cervicography plots cervical dilatation against time in labour. Since there is little cervical dilatation in the latent phase, its use is inappropriate, and cervicograms in the literature relate only to the active phase. There is an inductogram that plots Bishop Score against time. This was designed (as the name suggests) to monitor progress from the onset of purposeful uterine activity in labour induced by amniotomy and oxytocin titration. Whether it is appropriate to use it in the latent phase of spontaneous labour is speculative.

Cervicography will identify aberrant progress according to the limits set. Aberrant patterns do not correlate well with underlying pathology, and aetiologies must be sought by careful scrutiny of other clinical features. A 2-hour action line only gives a 50:50 chance of the woman needing an operative delivery, whether this be caesarean section or instrumental vaginal. (This statement is based on retrospective data; no prospective evaluation has been performed.)

*See Chapter 20, Routine intrapartum care: an overview.*

## 79. The following are of proven benefit with regard to preterm labour:

A. Oral metronidazole in women at high risk of preterm labour who are positive for bacterial vaginosis.                                                                    **True**

B. Treatment of asymptomatic bacteriuria with antibiotics.                               **True**

C. Hospitalization for bed rest for women at high risk.                                   **False**

D. Antibiotics for women presenting with threatened preterm labour with intact membranes.                                                                              **False**

E. Oral tocolysis in women at high risk of preterm labour.                                **False**

F. Antenatal treatment of group B *Streptococcus* (GBS).                                  **False**

In women with bacterial vaginosis at high risk for preterm labour, treatment with metronidazole reduces the risk of premature delivery by 60 per cent. Asymptomatic bacteriuria is associated with premature labour, and treatment reduces this risk. Bed rest in hospital for women at high risk of preterm labour increases the risks of early delivery. The ORACLE trial showed no evidence for the use of antibiotics in women with threatened preterm labour if membranes were intact. Oral tocolytics do not reduce the risk of preterm labour. There is some evidence that some classes of tocolytics – cyclo-oxygenase-2 (COX-2) inhibitors – may increase the risk if used as prophylaxis in high-risk women. Although GBS is problematic for many premature infants, there is no evidence that antenatal treatment reduces this risk. Studies have demonstrated problems with penicillin-resistant *Escherichia coli* in women treated aggressively antenatally for GBS.

*See Chapter 21, Preterm labour.*

## 80.  With regard to preterm labour:
A. The rate of severe handicap for infants delivered at 24–26 weeks is 25 per cent.    **True**
B. The risk of preterm labour is inversely proportional to cervical length.    **True**
C. Digital cervical length assessment is as clinically useful as ultrasound assessment.    **False**
D. Home uterine activity monitoring is ineffective in reducing the risk of preterm labour.    **True**
E. Tocolysis for threatened preterm labour reduces the risk of delivery within 48 hours.    **True**

Data from the UK EPIcure study demonstrated that 50 per cent of infants born at 24–26 weeks have some handicap, but only half of these were classed as severe. Studies of both high-risk and low-risk cohorts have shown that the incidence of preterm labour is directly related to cervical length, but that this is only accurate if measured ultrasonographically. Transvaginal ultrasound is the most accurate method. Home uterine activity monitoring in high-risk women has not been shown to be useful, possibly as there are no interventions to use if subclinical activity is detected. Tocolysis with beta-adrenergic agonists, oxytocin antagonists and calcium channel blockers all reduce the risk of delivery within 48 hours. Tocolytics used alone do not improve fetal outcome.
*See Chapter 21, Preterm labour.*

## 81.  With regard to pre-labour rupture of membranes (PROM) at term:
A. Ninety per cent of women will labour within 24 hours.    **False**
B. Ultrasound is not a useful primary test in establishing the diagnosis.    **True**
C. Women should be allowed to choose whether to wait or to undergo induction immediately as the outcomes are the same.    **True**
D. Women with known GBS colonization should be recommended induction without delay.    **True**
E. Women induced with prostaglandin are less likely to need Syntocinon in labour.    **False**

At term, 75 per cent of women will labour within 24 hours. Ultrasound evaluation of liquor volume is not helpful in establishing a primary diagnosis, but may be useful if labour has not ensued after 48 hours if the diagnosis remains unclear. The Canadian TERMPROM trial demonstrated no difference in outcomes whether induction was commenced immediately or delayed. This trial also demonstrated no difference in the need for Syntocinon regardless of whether prostaglandins were used as the first method of induction. Women with known GBS should commence intravenous antibiotics once PROM has been established and should be recommended immediate induction of labour.
*See Chapter 22, Pre-labour rupture of membranes.*

### 82. For women with preterm pre-labour rupture of membranes (PPROM):

A. Cervical length measurement is useful in predicting preterm labour.    **True**

B. The risk of placental abruption is approximately 5 per cent.    **True**

C. Single-course maternal steroid administration does not increase the risk of maternal infection.    **True**

D. Maternal steroid administration does not reduce the incidence of neonatal respiratory distress syndrome.    **False**

E. Antibiotic therapy improves neonatal mortality and morbidity rates.    **True**

Cervical length is a poor predictor of preterm labour once membranes have ruptured. As well as PPROM being a common sequela of antepartum haemorrhage, early membrane rupture carries a 5 per cent risk of subsequent abruption. However, this risk varies inversely with gestational age and is reportedly as high as 50 per cent below 24 weeks. Although neonates born after PPROM are reported to have lower incidences of respiratory distress syndrome when compared to neonates born preterm without PPROM, maternal steroids still appear to reduce the risk further. Maternal steroid administration as a single course does not increase the risk of maternal infection.

Erythromycin used for 10 days after PPROM is associated with a significant reduction (from 14.4 per cent to 11.2 per cent) in neonatal mortality and major morbidity.

*See Chapter 22, Pre-labour rupture of membranes.*

### 83. Planned induction of labour:

A. Should occur in less than 15 per cent of patients.    **True**

B. Should be performed before 41 weeks in cases of presumed fetal macrosomia.    **False**

C. In the presence of intact membranes, should involve prostaglandin administration regardless of the cervical status.    **True**

D. Should not be offered electively before 41 weeks' gestation.    **False**

E. Should not be offered to a patient who has previously been delivered by caesarean section.    **False**

There is no appropriate induction of labour rate in an unselected population. However, the WHO suggests that there is little improvement in maternal or fetal outcomes when levels of induction exceed 15 per cent. The management of macrosomia is contentious. There are no data to support induction of labour before 41 weeks to reduce the incidence of maternal or fetal problems for this indication. The guidelines of the RCOG and National Institute for Clinical Excellence (NICE) recommend induction of labour with prostaglandin as the first method, regardless of cervical status. Despite the knowledge that induction of labour in uncomplicated pregnancies is associated with an increased risk of caesarean section if performed before 41 weeks, it must be considered where there are compelling maternal or social reasons. A full discussion of the risks of induction of labour following caesarean section must take place. There is evidence that induction of labour in women with a uterine scar increases the risk of scar rupture and dehiscence. The magnitude of this risk remains small. Therefore, there will be occasions when induction of labour is considered for women with a prior caesarean section.

*See Chapter 25, Induction of labour.*

## 84.  Regarding induction of labour:

A. Uterine hyperstimulation secondary to prostaglandin administration is best treated
with tocolysis.                                                                                **True**

B. Women with PROM at term (>37 weeks) should be offered a choice of immediate
induction of labour or expectant management.                                                   **True**

C. Uterine rupture occurs more frequently among women undergoing a trial of vaginal
delivery following caesarean section in their previous pregnancy than among those
undergoing elective repeat caesarean delivery.                                                 **True**

D. Neonatal jaundice has been reported following the use of prostaglandins during
induction of labour.                                                                           **False**

E. Women who do not labour after an induction should be offered caesarean section.   **True**

Hyperstimulation with prostaglandin used for induction of labour is not uncommon.
Strategies involve washing out or removing the prostaglandin, use of tocolysis and urgent
delivery. Tocolysis is often effective. Intravenous or subcutaneous routes are best. Inhaled
administration is ineffective. The TERMPROM study demonstrated no difference in outcomes
between women randomized to either immediate or delayed augmentation following
spontaneous rupture of membranes at term. Where logistically feasible, it is recommended
that women be given a choice as to whether to wait or proceed immediately. The rates of
uterine rupture are approximately doubled when women undergo induction of labour with a
single prior caesarean section scar, compared to women delivered by elective caesarean
section. A small increase in the rate of neonatal jaundice has been reported in women who
receive Syntocinon in labour. This is not the case for prostaglandin administration. The
management of failed induction of labour must be individualized. Caesarean section must be
considered as an option and discussed with women.

*See Chapter 25, Induction of labour.*

## 85.  Cephalo-pelvic disproportion (CPD) in the absence of gross pelvic abnormality
    can be diagnosed by:

A. Ultrasound scan.                                                                            **False**

B. A maternal stature of less than 155 cm.                                                     **False**

C. Lateral X-ray pelvimetry.                                                                   **False**

E. Pelvic examination.                                                                         **False**

F. Trial of vaginal delivery.                                                                  **True**

Ultrasound cannot predict that a labour will be complicated by CPD. Ultrasound estimation
of fetal size is an imprecise tool, and the mechanism of labour is governed by more than just
fetal size. Although maternal short stature carries a higher risk of CPD, there is no size below
which this is always going to happen. Therefore maternal height alone cannot predict CPD. It
has been demonstrated that X-ray pelvimetry does not improve the ability to discriminate
between women who will or will not develop CPD. Pelvic examination is equally unhelpful.
Because labour is a dynamic process involving many different biomechanical factors, it is the
only method currently available to diagnose CPD properly.

*See Chapter 27, Poor progress in labour.*

## 86.  Regarding progress in labour:

A. A normal cervicometric curve is associated with a caesarean section rate of less than 5 per cent.                                                                    **True**

B. Primary dysfunctional labour occurs in 10 per cent of nulliparous labours.    **False**

C. In a case of secondary arrest, augmentation may be associated with uterine rupture.                                                                                  **True**

D. A supportive partner during labour will reduce the incidence of delivery by caesarean section.                                                                        **False**

E. Augmentation with Syntocinon in the latent phase is associated with a reduction in the incidence of operative deliveries.                                           **False**

So-called 'normal' progress in labour is associated with very high rates of vaginal delivery. This is at least in part because the 'normal' curves were initially based on the rates of progress in women who had actually achieved a vaginal delivery. Primary dysfunctional labour is the commonest labour pattern in nulliparous labours, affecting 26 per cent of all labours. Augmentation of labour in cases of secondary arrest in multigravidae may lead to uterine rupture. This is almost unheard of in nulliparous women. The data suggest that the presence of a supportive professional in labour reduces the risk of caesarean section; unfortunately, this effect does not hold true for partners. There are no data to suggest that augmentation with Syntocinon in the first stage of labour affects outcome. This is particularly so for the latent phase, where augmentation has been shown to be ineffective.

*See Chapter 27, Poor progress in labour.*

## 87.  With regard to electronic fetal monitoring:

A. In low-risk pregnancies, continuous monitoring in labour has been shown to improve long-term outcomes.                                                               **False**

B. An admission CTG should be performed for all women in labour.                  **False**

C. Continuous fetal monitoring increases intervention in labour.                  **True**

D. An abnormal CTG suggests acidosis in 50 per cent of fetuses.                   **False**

E. Maternal oxygen therapy should be given if the CTG is pathological.           **False**

Continuous electronic monitoring does not improve long-term outcomes, although less acidosis and fewer fits occur in continuously monitored fetuses. The CTG is a poor predictor of fetal acidosis. Even in the most pathological traces, only 50 per cent of fetuses will be acidotic. Admissions CTGs increase intervention in labour without improving outcomes if utilized for women with problem-free pregnancies. The use of CTGs continuously in labour increases intervention. This can be kept to a minimum by the use of fetal blood sampling where appropriate. Oxygen therapy is of no proven benefit and may be harmful if used for long periods.

*See Chapter 29, Fetal compromise in the first stage of labour.*

## 88.  The following are normal in the first stage of labour:

A. A scalp pH of 7.24.                                           **True**

B. A base excess of −13 mmol/L.                                  **False**

C. Baseline variability on the CTG of 5–10 bpm.                  **True**

D. A baseline on CTG of 155 bpm.                                 **True**

E. Variable decelerations on CTG.                                **False**

A scalp pH of 7.2 is 2 SD from the mean in the first stage of labour. A base excess of −12 mmol/L is also 2 SD from the mean. The NICE guideline suggests that normal baseline variability is 5–25 bpm, and a normal baseline is 110–160 bpm. Although variable decelerations are common, they are suspicious and must be managed in accordance with the clinical scenario.

*See Chapter 29, Fetal compromise in the first stage of labour.*

## 89.  A classical caesarean section:

A. Is performed through a midline sub-umbilical incision.        **False**

B. Has a higher incidence of postoperative pyrexia than a lower segment approach.   **True**

C. Is indicated in the presence of a placenta praevia at term.   **False**

D. Is the incision of choice in an HIV-positive woman.           **False**

A classical incision can be performed through a transverse incision; this has the advantages of improved cosmetic results, decreased analgesic requirements and less postoperative pulmonary compromise, and superior wound strength. There are few indications for a classical caesarean section, and these do not include HIV positivity. In most cases of placenta praevia, a lower segment incision is possible.

*See Chapter 31, Caesarean section.*

## 90.  Regarding caesarean section:

A. It may be performed for a competent woman against her will for the benefit of the fetus.                                                    **False**

B. The commonest indication for caesarean hysterectomy is uterine atony.   **True**

C. Vertical transmission of HIV may be reduced by 50 per cent.   **True**

D. The case fatality rate for all caesarean sections is eight times that for vaginal delivery.                                                  **False**

Full informed consent must always be obtained prior to operation; a caesarean section should never be performed in a competent woman against her will. The case fatality rate for all caesarean sections is five times that for vaginal delivery.

*See Chapter 31, Caesarean section.*

### 91. Regarding fetal surveillance in the second stage of labour:

A. Continuous electronic fetal monitoring is recommended.                    **False**
B. There is no role for fetal blood sampling.                                **False**
C. Ninety per cent of CTGs will show some abnormality.                       **True**
D. Accelerations on CTG are commonly present.                                **False**
E. Late decelerations are uncommon.                                          **True**

In pregnancies that have been problem free, and where labour has progressed normally without concern, intermittent auscultation is acceptable. National guidelines, such as those issued by the RCOG and the NICE, suggest auscultating the fetal heart rate every 5 minutes in the second stage. Usually this is for 60 seconds following a contraction, in order to detect significant decelerations. Where there is concern about fetal well-being and an easy delivery is not possible, a fetal blood sample should be taken to assess whether it is possible to wait for descent or rotation. This may especially be the case where a passive second stage will improve the chance of more straightforward delivery. Evaluation of second stage CTGs has shown that a normal baseline in combination with an absence of decelerations is seen in only one-quarter of second stage heart rate tracings. Additionally, many CTGs exhibit either no accelerations or poor variability, resulting in 90 per cent of all second stage CTGs showing some degree of abnormality. Late decelerations are uncommon, however, affecting only 5 per cent of CTGs.

*See Chapter 32, Fetal compromise in the second stage of labour.*

### 92. The following increase the incidence of acidosis in the second stage of labour:

A. Meconium staining of the liquor.                                          **True**
B. Active pushing.                                                           **True**
C. Routine use of maternal oxygen therapy.                                   **True**
D. The absence of accelerations in an otherwise normal CTG.                  **False**
E. Deep variable decelerations.                                              **True**

Meconium staining of the liquor at any stage in labour is associated with an increased risk of acidosis. Fetal scalp lactate increases in parallel with the length of active pushing in the second stage and there is a progressive fall in fetal pH. Passive second stage appears to be equivalent to late first stage in its effect on fetal pH. Maternal oxygen therapy may be helpful if used for a short period while other measures are instituted. The routine use of oxygen therapy in the second stage has been found to lead to an increase in newborn acidosis. Deep variable decelerations, with a drop in fetal heart rate of more than 70 bpm, are associated with a ten-fold increase in the risk of metabolic acidosis. Accelerations are not commonly present in the second stage and their absence if the remainder of the CTG is normal is unlikely to be associated with acidosis.

*See Chapter 32, Fetal compromise in the second stage of labour.*

## 93. Regarding shoulder dystocia:

| | |
|---|---|
| A. It affects approximately 1 per cent of all labours. | **True** |
| B. It carries a recurrence risk of 30 per cent. | **False** |
| C. It is commoner in obese women. | **True** |
| D. Twenty per cent of babies with an Erb's palsy will have long-term problems. | **False** |
| E. Erb's palsy can occur in babies delivered by caesarean section. | **True** |

The lack of a universally agreed definition for shoulder dystocia hampers any estimate of incidence. As a rough guide, approximately 1 per cent of deliveries are complicated by shoulder dystocia; overall recurrence risks are approximately 10–15 per cent. Fetal macrosomia is a recognized risk factor; it is commoner in obese women and in women with impaired glucose metabolism.

Erb's palsy is also relatively common. Fortunately, with early recognition, prompt physiotherapy and even neurosurgical treatment, most cases improve over time, leaving only 1–2 per cent of shoulder dystocia cases with long-term dysfunction. It is recognized that Erb's palsy can occur in infants delivered by caesarean section. It is therefore likely that the stretching of the fetal neck and impaction under the symphysis are responsible for some cases of Erb's palsy.

*See Chapter 33, Shoulder dystocia.*

## 94. The following manoeuvres are recommended for the management of shoulder dystocia:

| | |
|---|---|
| A. McRobert's. | **True** |
| B. Fundal pressure. | **False** |
| C. Suprapubic pressure. | **True** |
| D. Wood's screw. | **True** |
| E. Bilateral episiotomy. | **False** |

McRobert's manoeuvre involves hyperflexion of the maternal thighs onto the maternal abdomen, either by the mother herself or by a pair of assistants. It has been shown radiographically to flatten the lumbosacral curve and lessen any obstruction from the sacral promontory. The anterior shoulder will often release with this simple measure.

*See Chapter 33, Shoulder dystocia.*

Suprapubic pressure is often used simultaneously. The aim is to move the shoulders into the wider oblique diameter of the pelvis and force the anterior shoulder under the symphysis pubis. If simple rotation fails and the posterior shoulder is below the sacral promontory, Wood's screw manoeuvre should be attempted. This involves rotating the posterior shoulder through 180° so that it becomes the anterior shoulder. By simultaneously combining this with a degree of downward traction, the rotated shoulder remains within the pelvis and appears under the symphysis.

Fundal pressure simply increases the impaction of the shoulder against the symphysis. Episiotomy is required only to increase room to facilitate manoeuvres. It does not resolve the problem, and a bilateral episiotomy should not be necessary.

*See Chapter 33, Shoulder dystocia.*

## 95. The following have been shown to reduce the risk of second-degree perineal trauma in labour:

A. Standing or squatting rather than lying prone.     **False**

B. Perineal massage in nulliparae.        **True**

C. Allowing spontaneous delivery of the head rather than controlling delivery. **False**

D. Ventouse rather than forceps delivery.       **True**

E. Epidural analgesia.           **False**

The mother's position during the second stage has little influence on perineal trauma. Women should be allowed to adopt any position for delivery that they are comfortable with, provided delivery can be achieved safely.

In nulliparae, during the weeks before giving birth, perineal massage appears to protect against perineal trauma. The HOOP trial showed no difference in rates of perineal trauma whether the fetal head was allowed to deliver spontaneously or was controlled by the midwife. Ventouse delivery is associated with less perineal trauma than forceps. Epidural analgesia increases the risk of instrumental delivery and therefore carries an increased risk of perineal trauma.

*See Chapter 36, Perineal trauma.*

## 96. Perineal discomfort after delivery can be reduced by:

A. Using a non-locking suture of the vaginal epithelium.    **True**

B. Using interrupted rather than subcuticular sutures to the perineal skin. **False**

C. Using rapidly absorbable polyglactin sutures rather than standard polyglactin
 sutures.            **False**

D. Leaving the perineal skin approximated to within 0.5 cm but not closed. **True**

E. Cleaning the episiotomy or trauma with saline rather than antiseptic. **False**

A continuous non-locking suture of the vaginal epithelium appears to cause less discomfort than a continuous locked suture. Less perineal discomfort and dysaesthesia occurs if the perineal skin is sutured with a continuous subcuticular suture than with interrupted sutures, but leaving the skin edges approximated but not sutured is probably best. Standard Vicryl does not cause more discomfort than Vicryl Rapide, but is more likely to require removal. There is no evidence that cleaning of the perineum with antiseptic improves infection rates or alters rates of perineal pain.

*See Chapter 36, Perineal trauma.*

## 97. Regarding hypoxic–ischaemic encephalopathy (HIE):

A. It affects approximately 1 per cent of infants.                                    **False**

B. Neurological sequelae are common in infants with mild HIE.              **False**

C. A persistently depressed Apgar score is associated with poor outcomes.   **True**

D. Most cases of cerebral palsy are due to HIE during labour.               **False**

E. Magnetic resonance imaging (MRI) is a useful modality in the first 48 hours
   of life.                                                                  **False**

F. Renal failure is commonly associated with severe HIE.                    **True**

Hypoxaemic–ischaemic encephalopathy affects approximately 1 per 1000 infants. The outcome for infants with severe HIE is usually poor; however, infants with mild HIE usually have a good outcome and neurological sequelae are uncommon. A persistently low Apgar score is associated with poor outcomes. Although cerebral palsy may be caused by hypoxia in labour, most cases are due to antenatal insult. Not all babies with cerebral palsy demonstrate HIE at birth. The value of neuroimaging is limited in the first 24–48 hours of life. Evidence of lesions in the thalami and basal ganglia, focal infarctions and changes in periventricular white matter are usually seen after the first 48 hours of life. Their presence before this suggests an antenatal insult. Other organ involvement is common with severe HIE, including renal failure, disseminated intravascular coagulopathy and necrotizing enterocolitis.

*See Chapter 37, Perinatal asphyxia.*

## 98. The following are features consistent with cerebral palsy secondary to an intrapartum event:

A. Spastic diplegia.                              **False**

B. A sentinel event during labour.               **True**

C. An Apgar score of 8 at 5 minutes.             **False**

D. A cord artery pH of 7.1.                       **False**

E. Onset of fits at 24–48 hours of age.           **True**

The neurological sequelae with intrapartum HIE usually result in motor problems and spastic quadriplegia or dyskinetic cerebral palsy, not diplegia. A sentinel event may be identified as the cause during labour. Apgar scores are usually very depressed and the cord artery pH is generally very low (<7). Very early-onset fits suggest an antepartum cause, whereas fits at 24–48 hours are seen with intrapartum events.

*See Chapter 37, Perinatal asphyxia.*

**99. Physiologically, the following are important considerations when resuscitating the newborn infant:**

A. The ductus arteriosus closes within hours of birth.                                    **False**

B. Pulmonary vascular pressures are increased by excessive use of high-concentration oxygen.                                                                               **False**

C. Hypothermia is associated with a worse neurological outcome.            **False**

D. Restoration of blood volume should be the priority to ensure adequate tissue perfusion.                                                                                **False**

E. Surfactant synthesis is affected by factors such as temperature, pH and hypoxaemia.                                                                                 **True**

A basic understanding of the cardiovascular and respiratory changes the infant undergoes at birth can make a large difference to the outcome in neonatal resuscitation. The ductus arteriosus may 'shut' physiologically in that there is a reversal of the fetal right-to-left shunt after birth. However, it does not anatomically shut for several days after birth. This can lead to significant problems with shunting through the duct in sick infants. Oxygen is a very effective pulmonary vasodilator, hence its use helps reduce high pulmonary vascular pressures. Whilst hypothermia has been associated with increased morbidity in the newborn, there is no evidence to suggest this includes poor neurological outcome. Indeed, there is evidence to the contrary. In any resuscitation, the first priority is to establish an airway and ventilate the lungs.

*See Chapter 37, Perinatal asphyxia.*

**100. At birth, the following are important:**

A. Oropharyngeal suctioning is the first priority to aid the infant to establish respiration.                                                                            **False**

B. History taking prior to birth is unnecessary as the principles of ABC (airways, breathing and circulation) apply regardless.                                 **False**

C. Preparation includes the checking of equipment, organization of staff, clear roles for individuals, good communication and parental involvement.       **True**

D. Catheterization of the umbilical vein requires a Seldinger technique as it is a central vessel.                                                                      **False**

E. Most neonatal resuscitation practice is based on well-researched evidence.   **False**

Most infants will clear their own airway. Rushing in with oropharyngeal suctioning could be detrimental. The presence of thick meconium is an exception. Targeted history taking can make a profound difference to the outcome of resuscitation. Preparation and information aid resuscitation, for example the knowledge that a twin delivery is imminent changes the approach needed. The umbilical vein is easily accessible. Using a Seldinger technique is more likely to damage the vessel. Most resuscitation is based on 'best practice' rather than evidence-based studies.

*See Chapter 37, Perinatal asphyxia.*

**101. The Apgar score:**

A. Is an international scoring system used to help direct the resuscitation of a
neonate.                                                                          **True**
B. Consists of five components, including heart rate, respiratory effort, skin colour,
muscle tone and activity, and infant responsiveness.                              **True**
C. Is very useful at predicting an infant's long-term outlook.                    **False**
D. Is scored at 1 minute and 5 minutes after the birth of the whole child.        **True**
E. Is medico-legally an extremely important part of any resuscitation
documentation.                                                                    **False**

The Apgar score is an internationally recognized scoring system used to assess an infant's
condition shortly after birth. Although frequently used to help with the resuscitation, it
should be remembered that it has its limitations just like any other tool. Many workers have
tried to use the Apgar score to predict long-term outcome. At best, it gives a fairly crude idea
of outcome, with lower scores being associated with a worse outlook. The timing of the score
is open to debate. However, most clinicians take time zero as the moment at which the whole
baby is delivered from the mother. Medico-legally, it is much more important that an accurate
account of events be made rather than simply documenting an Apgar score.

*See Chapter 37, Perinatal asphyxia.*

**102. During the resuscitation of an infant:**

A. The airway can be best maintained by placing the head in the neutral position.   **True**
B. The first steps involve drying the infant to maintain body warmth and stimulate
the child to establish respiration.                                               **True**
C. Continual assessment of the infant's condition is mandatory.                   **True**
D. Bag-valve-mask ventilation is performed at a rate of 30–40 inflations per minute,
in contrast to ventilation via an endotracheal tube, which is performed at a rate
of 60 breaths per minute.                                                         **False**
E. Rescue breaths are more forceful, prolonged inflations used to help establish a
functional residual volume in the lungs.                                          **True**

These are a few of the basic principles of resuscitation in the newborn. Familiarity with basic
life support of the newborn should be mandatory for all health professionals involved in their
care. The rate of ventilation is not altered whether it be via a mask system or an endotracheal
tube.

*See Chapter 37, Perinatal asphyxia.*

## 103. With regard to resuscitation in the newborn:

A. Chest compressions at a rate of 120 per minute are more effectively achieved using the 'hands around the chest with the thumbs over the sternum' method as opposed to the use of two fingers placed over the sternum.   **False**

B. It is more important that the sternum is depressed a third of the antero-posterior diameter than that the rate of 120 compressions per minute is achieved when performing chest compressions.   **True**

C. The recommendation of high-concentration oxygen during resuscitation of the newborn is based on its associated protective effects on long-term lung damage.   **False**

D. Endotracheal adrenaline is as effective as intravascular adrenaline.   **False**

E. There is a medico-legal obligation to continue all resuscitative efforts for a minimum of 30 minutes without any signs of life before discontinuing care.   **False**

There is no evidence to show that chest compressions are better achieved using either two fingers over the sternum or both hands around the chest with the thumbs over the sternum. It is more important that the operator is proficient in one of these techniques. High-concentration oxygen is recommended as best practice. It makes sense to optimize oxygenation, thus improving oxygen delivery to vital organs. However, there is increasing concern about its use, especially in the preterm infant. Endotracheal adrenaline is not as effective as intravascular adrenaline.

The continuation of resuscitative efforts in the hopeless situation provokes many emotions. Most clinicians would advocate continuing for 15 minutes. After this, if there are still no signs of life, it is extremely unlikely to be successful and further resuscitative attempts are probably inappropriate.

*See Chapter 38, Neonatal resuscitation.*

## 104. When performing a newborn check, the following are important:

A. The examination must be performed after 24 hours of life.   **False**

B. A clicky hip suggests a dislocated hip requiring orthopaedic management.   **False**

C. The Mongolian blue spot is a birthmark that is unimportant and can be ignored.   **False**

D. Discussion of an infant's feeding pattern with the mother should be a standard part of the newborn examination.   **True**

E. A neonate that has not opened its bowels by 24 hours of life needs to be investigated for possible Hirschprung's disease.   **False**

Whilst it is not recommended to perform a newborn screening examination before 24 hours of age, due to the high incidence of false-positive and false-negative findings, this is not a hard and fast rule. Clicky hips are most likely to be due to lax ligaments around the joint and not dislocation, which is indicated by a 'clunk'. Mongolian blue spots are birthmarks found over the lumbosacral region. They should be documented in the infant records as they have been mistaken for bruising secondary to non-accidental injury. Most newborn infants open their bowels within the first 24 hours. However, it is not uncommon for them to delay until 48–72 hours of life. Those that have still not opened their bowels after this time need further investigation.

*See Chapter 39, Common neonatal problems.*

**105.  The following increase the risk of GBS infection in the newborn infant:**

A. History of a previous infant with GBS infection.                          **True**

B. Spontaneous onset of premature labour.                                    **True**

C. A positive urine culture for GBS in the mother during pregnancy.          **True**

D. Transient tachypnoea of the newborn following elective lower segment caesarean
   section.                                                                  **False**

E. Severe jaundice of the newborn presenting in the first 24 hours of life.  **False**

Transient tachypnoea of the newborn is probably due to excessive lung fluid. It resolves within the first few days of life. Severe jaundice in the first 24 hours may be secondary to sepsis, of which GBS is one cause; however, it is much more likely to be indicative of haemolysis due to Rhesus or ABO incompatibility.

*See Chapter 39, Common neonatal problems.*

**106.  These skin disorders are clinically significant in the newborn infant:**

A. Erythema toxicum neonatorum.                                              **False**

B. Traumatic cyanosis.                                                       **False**

C. Aplasia cutis.                                                            **True**

D. Flammeus naevus.                                                          **False**

E. Miliaria.                                                                 **False**

Erythema toxicum neonatorium is a benign rash, as is miliaria, which is due to blocked sweat glands. Flammeus naevus is a birthmark found over the forehead. It is more commonly referred to as the 'stork mark'. Traumatic cyanosis consists of multiple petechiae seen over the face and head. It often has a characteristic dusky appearance as well. However, it can be distinguished from true cyanosis, as the inside of the mouth and rest of the body are pink.

   Aplasia cutis is a skin defect seen over the scalp. It has the appearance of an injury with skin and hair loss. It occurs antenatally. The cause is unclear. It can be distinguished from acute scalp injuries at birth due to the appearance of the healed, rolled edge. It often requires plastic surgery at a later stage.

*See Chapter 39, Common neonatal problems.*

## 107. The following are true:

A. Erb's palsy involving cervical nerve roots C3 and C4 is associated with a good outcome. **False**

B. Hypothermia is associated with an increased risk of respiratory distress syndrome. **True**

C. Cephalhaematomas that enlarge further at a few weeks of age indicate further bleeding and require investigation. **False**

D. Sternomastoid tumours occur as a result of minor bleeding into the muscle and need physiotherapy to prevent shortening of the muscle as well as disturbance of visual development. **True**

E. Fracture of the clavicle from birth requires immobilization of the arm for 48 hours. **False**

Erb's palsy is due to damage to C5, 6 and 7. The enlargement of cephalhaematomas after a few weeks is usually secondary to breakdown of the clot, which then leads to absorption of water into the mass due to osmotic gradients. The haematoma is fluctuant and transient. The infant is well throughout this. Fractured clavicles need no treatment. Immobilizing the arm may be detrimental in the newborn as it can cause distress.

*See Chapter 39, Common neonatal problems.*

## 108. The following are commonly encountered in the newborn infant:

A. Infants born at term by breech extraction are at high risk of hypoglycaemia if they have not fed within the first 2–4 hours. **False**

B. Large bilateral hydroceles. **True**

C. An innocent heart murmur as indicated by a soft thrill and radiation to the apex. **False**

D. A deep-seated sacral dimple, the base of which is difficult to visualize. **True**

E. Umbilical granulomas. **False**

Breech extraction itself is not a risk factor for neonatal hypoglycaemia. An innocent murmur is indicated by a soft noise localized to the lower left sternal edge, with no radiation and varying in quality with positioning and respiration. A loud murmur with or without any other cardiac signs suggests a pathological cause until proven otherwise. The deep-seated sacral dimple in which the base is not easily seen is a great cause for anxiety. Fortunately, the bottom of most pits can be seen with a little perseverance. Umbilical granulomas do not present until a few weeks of life.

*See Chapter 39, Common neonatal problems.*

### 109. Amniotic fluid embolism:

| | |
|---|---|
| A. Occurs in up to 1 in 2000 pregnancies. | **False** |
| B. Is the third commonest cause of direct maternal death in the UK. | **False** |
| C. Occurs most commonly immediately postpartum. | **False** |
| D. Is associated with artificial rupture of membranes. | **True** |

Amniotic fluid embolism is a common cause of maternal death, complicating approximately 1 in 20 000 pregnancies and being the fifth most common cause of direct maternal death in the UK. It is believed that amniotic fluid and associated debris enter the circulation and cause an anaphylactoid-type reaction. Amniotic fluid embolism occurs most commonly in labour (70 per cent) and is associated with amniotomy in 78 per cent of cases. It is an obstetric emergency.

*See Chapter 41, Postpartum collapse.*

### 110. With regard to pulmonary embolism:

| | |
|---|---|
| A. It accounts for >50 per cent of all maternal deaths in the UK. | **False** |
| B. In pregnancy the risk is increased two-fold. | **False** |
| C. Antenatal presentation is most common. | **False** |
| D. It is associated with high body mass index. | **True** |

Pulmonary embolism is the most common cause of maternal death in the UK, being responsible (at least partially) for 33 per cent of maternal deaths. In the thrombogenic state of pregnancy, the risks are increased six-fold. The risks are further increased in pregnancies associated with:

operative delivery
increasing age
obesity
congenital or acquired thrombophilia
surgical procedures.

*See Chapter 41, Postpartum collapse.*

### 111. With regard to massive postpartum haemorrhage:

| | |
|---|---|
| A. It complicates 5 per cent of all pregnancies. | **False** |
| B. It is the third most common cause of direct maternal death in the UK. | **False** |
| C. Consumptive coagulopathy may worsen the prognosis. | **True** |
| D. If caused by uterine atony, it may be managed using a Rusch balloon. | **True** |

Massive obstetric haemorrhage is defined as blood loss of >1500 mL. The most common cause is postpartum haemorrhage, which is a major cause of maternal mortality. It occurs in 6.7 per 1000 maternities and is the sixth most common direct cause of maternal death in the UK. Management involves resuscitation of the mother, with restoration of circulating blood volume and the correction of disseminated intravascular coagulopathy. In severe uterine atony, the placement of a hydrostatic balloon into the uterine cavity may save the woman's life without redress to hysterectomy.

*See Chapter 42, Postpartum haemorrhage.*

### 112. Morbidly adherent and retained placenta:

A. Is associated with elevated serum aFP.                                    **True**

B. Is associated with elevated serum βhCG.                                   **True**

C. Is more common in women under the age of 35 years.                        **False**

D. Is more common in women who have placenta praevia.                        **True**

Placenta accreta has become more prevalent over the last 50 years and is a significant cause of massive postpartum haemorrhage, the incidence having increased ten-fold. A large cohort study from Taiwan indicated that risk factors for placenta accreta were:

   placenta praevia (OR 54.2, 95% CI 17.8–165.5)

   elevated maternal serum aFP (MSaFP) >2.5 multiple of the median (MoM) (OR 8.3, 95% CI 1.8–39.8)

   elevated βhCG (OR 3.9, 95% CI 1.5–9.9)

   maternal age >35 years (OR 3.2, 95% CI 1.1–9.5).

The complication was found to occur in 9.3 per cent of women with placenta praevia.

*See Chapter 42, Postpartum haemorrhage.*

### 113. In septic shock:

A. Two to three per cent of pregnant women die.                              **True**

B. The most common infective organisms in pregnancy are *Escherichia coli*.  **False**

C. Association with adult respiratory syndrome carries a mortality of 50 per cent.  **True**

D. There may be an association with systemic inflammatory response syndrome.  **True**

E. Administration of activated protein C may reduce mortality.               **True**

Pregnant women are usually fit and healthy. Only 0.4 per cent of pregnant women who develop bacteraemia go on to develop septic shock; 2–3 per cent of these die. In the last CEMD triennial report, the mortality associated with sepsis in pregnancy was 6.4 per million maternities. The most common infective organisms are *Streptococcus* Group A and B. Systemic inflammatory response syndrome is defined as being associated with any two of the following:

   temperature >38°C or <36°C

   respiratory rate >24 breaths/minute

   tachycardia >90 bpm

   leucocytosis >11 000/mm$^3$

   leucopenia <4000/mm$^3$.

*See Chapter 43, Postpartum pyrexia.*

**114. Common causes of sepsis in obstetric cases include:**
A. Chorioamnionitis.                                                    **True**
B. Intracerebral abscess.                                               **False**
C. Necrotizing fasciitis.                                               **True**
D. Pneumonia.                                                           **True**
E. Pancreatitis.                                                        **True**

Whereas an intracerebral abscess is an uncommon finding in pregnancy, the other precipitants are well recognized.
*See Chapter 43, Postpartum pyrexia.*

**115. Adverse changes in postnatal affect:**
A. Occur in >50 per cent of women.                                     **True**
B. Are morbid in 25 per cent of women.                                 **False**
C. Are associated with psychosis in 5 per cent of women.               **False**
D. Are more common in women who have experienced them in a previous pregnancy. **True**

Antenatal disturbances in mood or affect are usually due to pre-existing psychiatric conditions. More than 50 per cent of women suffer from postnatal 'blues'. The incidence of postnatal depression is 10–15 per cent and psychosis is relatively rare (0.1 per cent of women).
*See Chapter 44, Disturbed mood.*

**116. With regard to postnatal depression:**
A. It may be associated with pre-conceptual psychiatric illness.        **True**
B. It may be controlled by adjuvant oestrogen therapy.                  **True**
C. Tricyclic antidepressants are less effective than cognitive therapy. **False**
D. It may be monitored using the Edinburgh Score.                       **True**

Most drugs used to treat psychiatric disorders are relatively safe to use in pregnancy. The best treatment for postnatal depression appears to be cognitive–behavioural therapy, with the administration of antidepressants where necessary. However, a RCT has shown that fluoxetine is as effective as cognitive–behavioural therapy for the treatment of postnatal depression. Systematic reviews of two RCTs found progesterone therapy to be of no benefit, although oestrogen therapy decreased the severity of depression when used as adjuvant therapy. Cohort studies show that the Edinburgh Postnatal Depression Score is effective in detecting women at risk of postnatal mood disorders.
*See Chapter 44, Disturbed mood.*

### 117. Breastfeeding:

A. Occurs in >50 per cent of pregnancies in the UK.                                **True**
B. Is more common in women of lower socioeconomic class.                           **False**
C. Is commonly performed for more than 12 months postnatally.                      **False**

Approximately 62 per cent of women in England commence breastfeeding. It is much more common in women from social class 1 (90 per cent) than those in social class 5 (50 per cent). However, in the UK this will have fallen to approximately 29 per cent by 4 months postpartum. (This latter figure is corrected for both maternal age and the age at which full-time education was completed, and is therefore not directly comparable to the incidences quoted at delivery. Nevertheless it indicates a significant fall in the prevalence of breast-feeding with time.)

*See Chapter 45, Problems with breastfeeding.*

### 118. Mastalgia:

A. Is a common indication for cessation of breastfeeding.                          **True**
B. Is associated with delayed neonatal feeding.                                    **True**
C. Has an increased incidence in mothers using supplementary feeding.              **True**
D. Is relieved by the use of anti-inflammatory agents.                             **True**

Mastalgia is the most common reason for cessation of breastfeeding, especially when associated with engorgement. It is associated with:

    delayed initiation of feeding
    infrequent feeding
    time-limited feeds
    a late shift from colostrum to milk production
    a habit of supplementing feeds.

*See Chapter 45, Problems with breastfeeding.*

# GYNAECOLOGY

**119. In the normal development of the female reproductive tract:**

| | |
|---|---|
| A. The paramesonephric ducts develop at 10 weeks post-conception. | **False** |
| B. Anti-Müllerian hormone (AMH) leads to degeneration of the Müllerian ducts. | **True** |
| C. The paroophoron develops from the Wolffian ducts. | **True** |
| D. The myometrium develops from the Wolffian ducts. | **False** |
| E. The vaginal plate is derived from the urogenital sinus. | **True** |

The paramesonephric ducts (Müllerian ducts) develop during the sixth week of embryogenesis. During the same time the primitive sex cords form around the germ cells in the undifferentiated gonad. The fetal testes secrete AMH – also called Müllerian inhibiting substance (MIS) – which leads to the active regression of the Müllerian ducts. These also secrete androgens, leading to male external genital development and differentiation of the bilateral Wolffian ducts into the vas deferens, seminal vesicle and epididymis. The fetal ovaries are incapable of secreting androgens or AMH, therefore the female external genitalia develop with growth of the Müllerian ducts and regression of the Wolffian ducts. At week 8–10, the pelvic Müllerian ducts have fused, and subsequent breakdown of their medial walls leads to a single tube. This becomes the upper vagina, cervix and uterine epithelium and glands. The surrounding mesenchymal tissue develops into the myometrium and stroma.

*See Chapter 46, Normal and abnormal development of the genitalia.*

**120. Congenital adrenal hyperplasia:**

| | |
|---|---|
| A. Presents classically as neonatal hypernatraemia. | **False** |
| B. Presents classically as a feminized XY neonate. | **False** |
| C. Causes absolute infertility. | **False** |
| D. Leads to high circulating concentrations of testosterone. | **True** |
| E. Requires mineralocorticoid replacement. | **True** |

Congenital adrenal hyperplasia is an autosomal recessive disorder that causes a deficiency of cortisol. This leads to hyperplasia of the adrenal gland and the subsequent production of excessive androgens. These high circulating androgen levels lead to masculinizing effects at the external female genitalia, and ambiguous genitalia or normal-looking male genitalia at birth. The lack of cortisol is potentially life threatening to the neonate, as deficiency leads to neonatal hyponatraemia through the loss of salt. Females with congenital adrenal hyperplasia have the potential for fertility later in life, due to the fact that the XX fetus initially develops the ovary, uterus, cervix and upper vagina before the androgens can have their masculinizing effect. Management aims to correct the cortisol deficiency and excess androgen production.

*See Chapter 46, Normal and abnormal development of the genitalia.*

**121. The following statements refer to girls with congenital adrenal hyperplasia:**

A. The usual karyotype is 46XY.                                                    **False**

B. Most cases are due to a deficiency of the 21-hydroxylase enzyme.                **True**

C. Müllerian structures fail to develop in utero.                                  **False**

D. Poor compliance with treatment leads to raised levels of 17-alpha
   hydroxyprogesterone.                                                            **True**

E. Treated females have fertility rates that are similar to those of unaffected women. **False**

The Müllerian structures develop in utero to form the uterus, cervix and upper vagina. This allows females with this condition the potential (although reduced) for fertility. The diagnosis of congenital adrenal hyperplasia is made on the increased levels of 17-alpha hydroxyprogesterone; therefore this makes an excellent marker of poor compliance.

*See Chapter 47, Karyotypic abnormalities.*

**122. When compared to women with a normal karyotype, women with Turner's syndrome (45X) have an increased incidence of the following medical conditions:**

A. Ovarian carcinoma.                                                              **False**

B. Hypertension.                                                                   **True**

C. Diabetes.                                                                       **True**

D. Cirrhosis of the liver.                                                         **False**

E. Deafness.                                                                       **True**

Turner's syndrome is the commonest chromosomal abnormality occurring in females; it affects 1 in 2000 live-born girls. Those affected have normal intelligence, although they may have various structural abnormalities, including web neck, renal agenesis, cardiac malformations and eye deformities. It is also associated with many long-term health issues, including premature ovarian failure (normally prior to the onset of puberty), hypertension, diabetes and sensorineural deafness. Osteoporosis is common in girls with Turner's syndrome, as an effect of oestrogen deficiency. Red/green colour blindness is also more common.

*See Chapter 47, Karyotypic abnormalities.*

### 123. Central precocious puberty:

A. Follows a premature suppression of pituitary luteinizing hormone (LH) and follicle-stimulating hormone (FSH) secretion due to activation of ovarian steroid synthesis.                                                        **False**

B. Should be investigated with cranial imaging techniques.                 **True**

C. Is frequently seen in girls with Turner's syndrome.                     **False**

D. Is frequently accompanied by a cessation of growth.                     **False**

E. Is frequently preceded by initiation of breast development.             **True**

Central precocious puberty is more common in females than in males. Investigations for those patients who present with suspected precocious puberty should include oestradiol, FSH and LH levels. These would be expected to be elevated into the normal female physiological ranges. Thyroid function tests should also be performed, as primary hypothyroidism can cause precocious puberty. An ultrasound of the pelvis should be arranged to exclude ovarian pathology. There are numerous brain pathologies that can cause precocious puberty, including tumours, trauma, infection and congenital malformations, and cranial imaging is indicated. Girls with Turner's syndrome have delayed puberty, due to the premature ovarian failure that is more common in this group of women. In most cases, breast development occurs prior to the onset of other characteristics.

*See Chapter 48, Menarche and adolescent gynaecology.*

### 124. In pubertal delay:

A. Elevated plasma concentrations of LH and FSH suggest a readily reversible cause. **False**

B. A 45XO karyotype suggests that the uterus has not developed.            **False**

C. Steroids can be given to induce breast development.                     **True**

D. Low concentrations of gonadotrophins are associated with excessive exercise. **True**

E. Bone age is retarded in constitutional delayed puberty.                 **True**

The presence of both high LH and high FSH suggests failure of gonadal development. The most common cause for this condition is Turner's syndrome, but it also occurs in pure gonadal dysgenesis. Other non-genetic causes include damage to the ovaries by irradiation, surgery, chemotherapy or infection. None of these causes is readily reversible. Turner's syndrome is associated with normal female genital development. Incremental doses of oestradiol (initially at 2 µg, increasing every 6 months to 20 µg) should be used to initiate breast development. Examination of bone age will demonstrate delay when compared to chronological age.

*See Chapter 48, Menarche and adolescent gynaecology.*

## 125. With regard to the human ovary:

A. The primordial follicles are embedded in the medulla.                    **False**

B. The maximum size of the primordial follicle pool is attained at birth.   **False**

C. Ovulation does not occur in utero.                                       **True**

D. Similar to the testis, the ovary originates from a coelomic projection known as the gonadal ridge.                                                         **True**

E. The hilar cells are differentiated cells that form the major source of ovarian peptide hormones.                                                            **False**

The primordial follicles are embedded in the stromal cells of the inner part of the cortex. The maximum size of the primordial follicle pool is attained at 6–8 weeks and from then onwards continuous rapid loss takes place. However, the loss of the follicles slows down after birth and occurs only as a result of follicular development followed by atresia. Follicular development occurs in utero; however, ovulation does not occur. Both the testes and ovaries develop from the gonadal ridge and pass through a stage of undifferentiated gonads. The hilar cells are undifferentiated cells that have the potential of steroidogenesis.

*See Chapter 49, Ovarian and menstrual cycles.*

## 126. In an ovulatory cycle:

A. Usually only one follicle develops every cycle.                          **False**

B. Both oestrogen and inhibin B are produced by the lead follicle.          **True**

C. Ovulation occurs 24–36 hours post-LH surge.                              **True**

D. The LH triggers the completion of the first mitotic division, resulting in the production of the first polar body.                                           **False**

E. Follicular development is dependent on the gonadotrophins throughout the cycle. **False**

Cohorts of follicles develop during the cycle; however, usually one known as the dominant follicle reaches the antral stage and ovulation. The LH surge triggers the completion of the first meiotic division (not mitotic). The follicular development in the beginning of the cycle is independent of gonadotrophins, during which time the follicles acquire FSH receptors and the one that acquires most receptors becomes the dominant follicle.

*See Chapter 49, Ovarian and menstrual cycles.*

### 127. Condoms:

| | |
|---|---|
| A. Have the additional benefit of reducing sexually transmitted diseases, including human immunodeficiency virus (HIV) disease. | **True** |
| B. Have a higher failure rate in circumcized men. | **False** |
| C. Have a reduced effectiveness in the presence of oestradiol creams. | **True** |
| D. Have a reduced effectiveness in the presence of K-Y jelly. | **True** |
| E. Have a quoted contraceptive efficacy of 3–23 per 100 woman-years. | **True** |

Condoms are a widely accessible form of reversible contraception. They are normally made from fine latex rubber; however, latex-free condoms are available for those with a latex allergy. Condoms are an effective method of reducing all sexually transmitted diseases. The published efficacy of condoms ranges from 3 to 23 per 100 woman-years. Most manufacturers advise against the use of additional creams and lubricants, as there is a theoretical risk of damaging the integrity of the latex in the condom.

*See Chapter 50, Contraception, sterilization and termination of pregnancy.*

### 128. With regard to laparoscopic clip sterilization:

| | |
|---|---|
| A. There is a failure rate of approximately 0.5 per cent. | **True** |
| B. Most deaths are due to anaesthetic complications. | **True** |
| C. The procedure should not be performed during menstruation. | **False** |
| D. All women should be counselled that male sterilization is a safer alternative. | **True** |
| E. Surgical emphysema is a recognized complication. | **True** |

Female sterilization involves the blockage of both fallopian tubes with either clips or rings. The failure rate for this procedure is quoted as 1:200. Although the procedure can be performed at any time during the female cycle, pregnancy needs to be excluded if the woman's period is late or she suspects that she might be pregnant. Male sterilization (vasectomy) is safer and equally effective as a method of contraception, and therefore all women should be aware that this is an alternative. Laparoscopy has a major complication rate of 5.7/100 000 procedures and a mortality rate of 4/100 000 procedures. Anaesthetic complications are the most common cause of death during laparoscopic sterilization.

*See Chapter 50, Contraception, sterilization and termination of pregnancy.*

## 129. With regard to the normal menstrual cycle:

A. The pulsatile release of gonadotrophin-releasing hormone (GnRH) increases in the luteal phase of the cycle.    **False**

B. The oestrogen surge precedes the LH surge by 12 hours.    **True**

C. Oestrogen receptor (ER) and progesterone receptor (PR) expression is maximal in the late luteal phase.    **False**

D. Ovulation occurs approximately 32 hours after the LH surge.    **True**

E. The number of endometrial leucocytes varies over the menstrual cycle.    **True**

In the normal menstrual cycle, GnRH is released in a pulsatile manor; however, the rate of this release varies between the follicular and luteal phases. In the follicular phase, GnRH pulses are released every 60–90 minutes; in the luteal phase, this release slows to every 120–180 minutes. Both the ER and PR are localized within the nuclei of the target cells, with maximal stromal and glandular expression occurring in the late follicular phase. The leucocyte population within the endometrium consists mainly of macrophages and lymphocyctes. The type and number of these cells vary over the menstrual cycle.

*See Chapter 51.1, Endometrial function.*

## 130. Uterine fibroids:

A. Are present in up to 25 per cent of women of reproductive age.    **True**

B. Are the most common site of leiomyosarcoma development.    **False**

C. If small and submucous, are unlikely to be associated with menorrhagia.    **False**

D. Can be accurately located on pelvic ultrasound.    **True**

E. If palpable abdominally, should be removed.    **False**

Uterine fibroids are present in approximately 25 per cent of the female population of reproductive age. This increases to 40 per cent in women who have a confirmed blood loss of >200 mL. Smoking and the long-term use of the oral contraceptive pill and Depo-Provera® are associated with a reduced risk. Only 10–15 per cent of leiomyosarcomas develop from uterine fibroids; the remainder occur spontaneously within the myometrium. Pelvic ultrasound (either transabdominal or transvaginal) should be the first choice of investigation and it should be possible to document the size and position of the fibroids. The initial treatment should be conservative, and surgery should only be used after medical therapy has failed.

*See Chapter 51.2, Uterine fibroids and menorrhagia.*

**131. Recognized side effects of danazol include:**

A. Weight gain.                                    **True**

B. Vaginal dryness.                                **True**

C. Increase in breast size.                        **False**

D. Acne.                                           **True**

E. Hirsutism.                                      **True**

Danazol is an isoxazol derivative of 17-alpha ethyl testosterone. Its side effects are dose dependent and are related to the hypo-oestrogenic environment that it creates in combination with its androgenic properties. Danazol inhibits ovarian steroidogenesis by inhibiting the mid-cycle LH/FSH surge. It also has the effect of increasing the free testosterone concentration via a reduction in sex hormone-binding globulin (SHBG). The most common side effects are weight gain, fluid retention, fatigue, decreased breast size, acne, oily skin, growth of facial hair, atrophic vaginitis, hot flushes and muscle cramps. At higher doses it also causes an irreversible deepening of the voice. Danazol also has metabolic effects that include increased low-density lipoproteins (LDL) and a reduction in the high-density lipoproteins (HDL) and serum cholesterol.

*See Chapter 51.2, Uterine fibroids and menorrhagia.*

**132. In the management of menorrhagia:**

A. Norethisterone is the treatment of choice for reducing menstrual loss in simple
   menorrhagia.                                    **False**

B. Oestrogen-impregnated intrauterine devices are useful for reducing menstrual
   loss.                                           **False**

C. Hysteroscopy allows visualization of the ovarian surfaces.    **False**

D. Endometrial sampling on day 7 of the cycle will usually reveal proliferative
   endometrium.                                    **True**

E. GnRH agonists are a cost-effective alternative to the oral contraceptive pill.    **False**

Cyclical progestogens were used in the past, although current evidence does not support their use for simple menorrhagia when given only during the luteal phase of the cycle. However, there is limited evidence to support the use of cyclical progestogens for the control of anovulatory dysfunctional bleeding. Progesterone-impregnated intrauterine devices such as the Mirena® coil have proved excellent treatment modalities for the management of women with menorrhagia. The continuous exposure of the endometrium to progestagen induces progressive atrophy, with reduction of menstrual bleeding by more than 80 per cent after 3–6 months and by more than 90 per cent at 12 months. Hysteroscopy is only of value in assessing the endometrial cavity. In the normally ovulating woman, the endometrium has a proliferative pattern during the follicular phase, becoming secretory under the influence of post-ovulatory progesterone. GnRH agonists are contraceptive but far more costly than the combined oral contraceptive pill (COCP).

*See Chapter 51.3, Heavy and irregular menstruation.*

### 133.  The following relate to dysmenorrhoea:

A. Childbirth has a curative effect on secondary dysmenorrhoea.                    **False**

B. Women who have smoked for more than 10 years have an increased risk of
dysmenorrhoea.                                                                     **True**

C. Pain prior to menstruation suggests pelvic inflammatory disease (PID).          **False**

D. In secondary dysmenorrhoea, laparoscopy should be considered if a trial of
therapy is unsuccessful.                                                           **True**

E. The contraceptive pill is of value in its treatment.                            **True**

Childbirth has the effect of improving primary dysmenorrhoea. In PID, the pain usually occurs in the days following menstruation. Women who have smoked for 10–20 years have an approximately six-fold relative risk of developing dysmenorrhoea. Unless the history and examination are suggestive of pathology, trial of therapy is indicated. However, if this is unsuccessful, the patient requires further investigation. This investigation of choice would be laparoscopy.

The COCP is often the treatment of choice for women complaining of dysmenorrhoea who require an effective method of contraception. The mechanism of action appears to be a reduction in the contractility of the uterine myometrium.

*See Chapter 51.4, Dysmenorrhoea.*


### 134.  With regard to endometriosis:

A. It is associated with unruptured luteinized follicle.                           **False**

B. The severity of disease is determined by the American Fertility Score.          **True**

C. It can be treated with 200 mg danazol daily.                                    **True**

D. The results of medical treatment are poor compared to those of surgery.         **False**

E. It cannot occur de novo after sterilization.                                    **False**

Although associated with subfertility, the precise cause in endometriosis, particularly mild endometriosis, remains unknown. The American Fertility Score is particularly useful in comparative studies and to assess the results of the treatment. A dose of 200 mg of danazol may well be as effective as larger doses and there is evidence that amenorrhoea is not required. Results of medical treatment are good, particularly with the use of GnRH analogues. It is generally accepted that endometriotic tissue reaches the pelvis by retrograde menstruation; therefore it cannot occur de novo after sterilization.

*See Chapter 51.5, Endometriosis and gonadotrophin releasing hormone analogues.*

### 135. The diagnosis of adenomyosis requires:

A. A myometrial thickness of 2.5 cm or more.                                      **False**

B. Islands of endometrial glands without stroma in the myometrium.                **False**

C. Accompanying endometriosis elsewhere in the pelvis.                            **False**

D. Extension of the endometrial glands and stroma in the myometrium with adjacent
   smooth muscle hyperplasia.                                                     **True**

E. Subserosal disease near the uterine surface.                                   **False**

The incidence of adenomyosis is unknown; however, it is present in 15–30 per cent of hysterectomy specimens. Adenomyosis should be regarded as distinct from endometriosis in terms of its epidemiology, being most common in parous middle-aged women. Although histologically both seem to have a common origin, the two conditions do not normally co-exist. Most women who have adenomyosis present with a history of menorrhagia and dysmenorrhoea. Transvaginal ultrasound (TVUS) has been recommended as the first investigation. Various ultrasound characteristics have been suggested to be diagnostic of adenomyosis, these include diffuse echogenicity, myometrial cysts, poor definition of the endometrial border and asymmetric thickening of the myometrium. However, TVUS lacks specificity, in particular in distinguishing adenomyosis from fibroids.

*See Chapter 51.6, Adenomyosis.*

### 136. With regard to premenstrual syndrome:

A. It is a common clinical phenomenon affecting 40 per cent of the female
   population.                                                                    **False**

B. The symptoms occur at a time of relative progesterone deficiency.             **False**

C. It is not relieved by the end of menstruation.                                **False**

D. Evening primrose oil is effective at relieving the symptoms.                  **False**

E. Suppression of ovulation with transdermal oestrogen and progesterone for
   endometrial protection is an effective treatment.                             **True**

Premenstrual syndrome (PMS) is a cluster of menstrually related symptoms that include mood swings, tension, anger, irritability, headache, breast discomfort, bloating, increased appetite and food cravings. More than 90 per cent of women have at least one PMS symptom, which by definition is always cyclical. PMS symptoms always occur after ovulation and therefore are due to progesterone excess rather than deficiency. The use of progestogens in the treatment of PMS is analogous to down-regulation. Evening primrose oil is effective in reducing cyclical mastalgia; however, it has not been shown to have any benefit for the other symptoms of PMS. Transdermal oestradiol has been used in ovulation suppressive doses in combination with cyclical luteal phase progestogen for the management of severe PMS and has an overall satisfaction at 8 months of 50 per cent.

*See Chapter 51.7, Premenstrual syndrome.*

### 137. When investigating an infertile couple:

A. Routine hysteroscopy should be carried out.                                              **False**

B. A serum progesterone level >10 nmol/L on cycle day 21 is indicative of ovulation. **False**

C. Laparoscopy and dye hydrotubation is more informative of uterine cavity
   abnormality than hysterosalpingography.                                             **False**

D. Urinary LH detection using a commercially available test kit is diagnostic of
   ovulation.                                                                          **False**

E. A routine cervical smear should be included in the investigation of infertility.    **False**

There is no evidence that routine hysteroscopy offers any advantages in the investigation of the female partner's infertility unless a uterine factor is suspected from the patient's history or hysterosalpingogram (HSG). A serum progesterone level >30 nmol/L on cycle day 21 is indicative of ovulation in a 28-day cycle. Laparoscopy and tubal patency testing is more informative than HSG with regard to examining the peritoneal surface of the pelvic organs but lacks the information obtained via HSG about the uterine cavity. Urinary LH detection kits can detect LH surge, which does not necessarily mean ovulation. Evidence of an up-to-date negative cervical smear test is important for patients undergoing infertility investigations.

*See Chapter 52.2, Female infertility.*

### 138. In the management of female infertility:

A. Three cycles of superovulation and intrauterine insemination result in a better
   pregnancy rate compared to one in-vitro fertilization (IVF) cycle in patients with
   unexplained infertility.                                                            **True**

B. Ectopic pregnancy rates are similar between IVF and gamete intrafallopian transfer
   (GIFT) in patients with unexplained infertility.                                    **False**

C. Tubal surgery for hydrosalpynx results in pregnancy in more than 50 per cent
   of cases.                                                                           **False**

D. Infertile patients with mild endometriosis should be given long-term GnRH agonist
   treatment while awaiting IVF treatment.                                             **False**

E. Salpingectomy in patients with tubal factor infertility undergoing IVF improves the
   pregnancy rates.                                                                    **True**

Ectopic pregnancy rates are higher with GIFT in unexplained infertility than with IVF. Surgery for hydrosalpynx only results in pregnancy in about 20 per cent of cases. There is no evidence that medical treatment of endometriosis prior to IVF treatment improves the outcome. However, unless medically indicated to control symptoms, the administration of GnRH agonist is of no particular value. Salpingectomy of a hydrosalpynx that is visible on ultrasound scan offers better results with IVF treatment.

*See Chapter 52.2, Female infertility.*

## 139.  Regarding male factor investigations:

A. Semen analysis should be performed before investigations of the female partner.    **False**

B. Testing for anti-sperm antibodies should be carried out routinely.    **False**

C. The ratio of normal to abnormal sperm morphology is a sensitive marker of male fertility.    **False**

D. Testicular examination is ideally carried out in the supine position.    **False**

E. Ten per cent of azoospermic and severely oligozoospermic men are carriers of the cystic fibrosis gene.    **True**

Semen analysis should be the starting point in investigating the male partner. However, concurrent investigations of the female partner should also be undertaken, but with invasive testing of tubal patency being deferred until the results of other tests are available. Routine checking for anti-sperm antibodies has not been recommended in the Royal College of Obstetricians and Gynaecologists' (RCOG) guidelines. The value of the ratio of the normal to abnormal spermatozoa with regard to the likelihood of achieving a pregnancy has been controversial and a normal range has not been established for the fertile population.

*See Chapter 52.3, Male infertility.*

## 140.  Regarding the management of male factor infertility:

A. Varicocelectomy is effective in improving male fertility when associated with severe oligospermia.    **True**

B. Bromocriptine is useful in treating sperm abnormalities and sexual dysfunction in infertile men.    **False**

C. Patients with Kallmann's syndrome can be treated effectively with gonadotrophins.    **True**

D. Sperm washing and intrauterine insemination are effective in treating asthenospermia due to anti-sperm antibodies.    **False**

E. Obtaining and freezing a sperm sample from the epididymis is essential during vasectomy reversal as the procedure has a high failure rate.    **False**

Surgical excision of a clinically apparent varicocele is effective in cases of severe oligozoospermia. Bromocriptine is useful in treating sexual dysfunction in men with hyperprolactinaemia. However, its value in treating sperm abnormalities is doubtful.

Kallmann's syndrome is associated with hypogonadotrophic hypogonadism, hence the use of exogenous gonadotrophin treatment in these cases. Sperm washing has not been shown to improve the pregnancy rates of the partners of men with high titres of anti-sperm antibodies. Retrieving and freezing sperm during the reversal of vasectomy procedures is considered good practice in case of failure. Reversal of vasectomy has a high success rate with regard to rejoining the vas; however, the pregnancy rates are usually lower due to the development of anti-sperm antibodies.

*See Chapter 52.3, Male infertility.*

## 141. The following statements are true:

A. IVF is a suitable first-line option for treating all types of infertility.  **False**

B. Optional transfer of two instead of three embryos does not reduce the pregnancy rate.  **True**

C. Transferring two or three embryos has the same twin pregnancy rates.  **False**

D. Not proceeding with embryo transfer prevents late-onset ovarian hyperstimulation syndrome (OHSS).  **False**

E. Recombinant FSH offers a higher pregnancy rate compared to high-purity urinary gonadotrophins.  **True**

In-vitro fertilization is a suitable treatment for all types of infertility but not as a first line. The transfer of two embryos compared to three does not result in a reduction of the pregnancy rate. However, the transfer of three does result in a high rate of multiple pregnancies. Not proceeding with embryo transfer reduces the severity but not the incidence of late-onset OHSS. More recent reports suggest that recombinant FSH is associated with higher pregnancy rates than urine-derived gonadotrophins.

*See Chapter 52.4, Assisted reproduction.*

## 142. With regard to OHSS:

A. It can lead to hypovolaemia and haemoconcentration in severe cases.  **True**

B. Mild and moderate cases can be treated at home.  **True**

C. Albumin replacement is essential for most cases.  **False**

D. Paracentesis should be avoided at all costs.  **False**

E. It is commoner in polycystic ovarian syndrome (PCOS) and lean patients.  **True**

Albumin replacement is only indicated if a significant drop in serum albumin occurs. Paracentesis is indicated if the patient's breathing is compromised or if the patient is very uncomfortable. The procedure should be carried out under ultrasound guidance to avoid any damage to the enlarged ovaries.

*See Chapter 52.4, Assisted reproduction.*

### 143.  Polycystic ovarian syndrome:

A. Is associated with LH hypersecretion.                                     **True**

B. Is associated with low TSH levels.                                        **False**

C. Typically presents with primary amenorrhoea.                              **False**

D. Is associated with increased production of dehydroepiandrosterone sulphate
   (DHEAS), an adrenal androgen.                                             **True**

E. Is associated with markedly elevated serum prolactin.                     **False**

Polycystic ovarian syndrome is the presence of polycystic ovaries and a particular cluster of symptoms that include amenorrhoea, oligomenorrhoea, hirsutism, anovulation and other signs of androgen excess such as acne. Biochemically it is associated with high LH concentrations and a low or normal FSH level. Despite there being many dramatic biochemical changes with PCOS, there is no alteration in the thyroid-stimulating hormone levels. Only 10 per cent of women present with primary amenorrhoea. PCOS typically presents with secondary amenorrhoea and is the most common cause of anovulatory infertility. Testosterone is the major circulating androgen in females. However, DHEAS is synthesized to a lesser extent, and is almost exclusively synthesized in the adrenal glands. It is used as marker of abnormal adrenal steroid metabolism and 50 per cent of women with PCOS demonstrate elevated levels. It is also associated with a decrease in the SHBG levels, therefore increasing the free androgen concentration. Ten per cent of women with PCOS have elevated prolactin levels; however, these are always <1000 IU/mL.

*See Chapter 53, Polycystic ovarian syndrome.*

### 144.  The following are inconsistent with a diagnosis of PCOS:

A. A regular 28-day cycle.                                                   **False**

B. Normal ovarian morphology on ultrasound scan.                            **True**

C. LH:FSH ratio <2:1.                                                        **False**

D. Normal body mass index.                                                  **False**

E. Rapidly progressive virilization.                                        **True**

Women with PCOS classically present with irregular cycles. The diagnosis is made on several criteria, including the presence of abnormal ovarian morphology. The diagnostic criterion of ten discrete follicles of <10 mm, usually peripherally arranged around an enlarged, hyperechogenic central stroma, is still held today. The LH:FSH ratio is in the order of >3:1; however, this is not essential for the diagnosis. Approximately 25 per cent of women with PCOS are obese. Rapidly progressive virilization is uncommon, as this usually reflects high levels of free testosterone.

*See Chapter 53, Polycystic ovarian syndrome.*

### 145. With respect to the management of anovulatory infertility in a woman with PCOS:

A. Weight reduction is ineffective in improving fertility. **False**

B. Ultrasound follicular tracking is not necessary if clomiphene citrate is used for fewer than 12 cycles. **False**

C. Use of clomiphene citrate for fewer than 12 cycles has been shown to be associated with an increased risk of ovarian cancer. **False**

D. Tamoxifen is an alternative to clomiphene citrate. **True**

E. The recommended duration of use of gonadotrophin therapy is 6–12 months. **False**

In women with PCOS, moderate obesity is associated with reduced ovulation. The loss of as little as 10 per cent of the body weight may result in a return to regular ovulation. Ovulation induction with clomiphene citrate should be undertaken in circumstances in which there is access to ultrasound follicle tracking. There is no evidence to suggest an increased risk of ovarian cancer when clomiphene is used for less than 12 cycles, with the current recommendation being not to exceed 6 months of continuous therapy. Tamoxifen is a drug that is similar in structure and function to clomiphene. It appears to be as effective as clomiphene at ovulation induction, although the trials are few and small.

*See Chapter 53, Polycystic ovarian syndrome.*

### 146. With respect to the management of anovulatory infertility in a woman PCOS:

A. Laparoscopic ovarian drilling is more effective than gonadotrophin therapy in women who are clomiphene resistant. **False**

B. Laparoscopic ovarian drilling is associated with an increased risk of multiple pregnancy. **False**

C. Laparoscopic ovarian drilling is associated with OHSS. **False**

D. Ultrasound follicular tracking is unnecessary in women treated with laparoscopic ovarian drilling. **True**

E. Laparoscopic ovarian drilling is associated with a normalization of LH levels. **True**

Laparoscopic drilling of the ovaries has been demonstrated to be as effective as gonadotrophin therapy in the induction of ovulation in women with PCOS. The advantages of ovarian drilling include a lower incidence of multiple gestations and the absence of hyperstimulation. The risks involved in this form of treatment are mainly associated with the operation. These include the risks of laparoscopy and anaesthesia and diathermy damage to adjacent tissues.

*See Chapter 53, Polycystic ovarian syndrome.*

## 147. The following are long-term consequences of PCOS:

A. Increased mortality from cardiovascular disease.          **False**
B. Increased risk of ovarian cancer.                         **True**
C. Increased risk of endometrial cancer.                     **True**
D. Increased risk of insulin-dependent diabetes mellitus.    **True**
E. Increased risk of osteoporosis.                           **False**

Polycystic ovarian syndrome is associated with several long-term health issues. There is 2.5-fold increase in the incidence of ovarian cancer when compared to control women. Endometrial cancer has a five-fold increase in incidence in women with PCOS, possibly due to the effect that unopposed oestrogens have on the endometrium in women with irregular cycles. Despite the significant effects that PCOS has on female steroid metabolism, bone density appears to be unaffected because of possible supernormal mineralization with androgens. As well as the effects on steroid metabolism, PCOS is also associated with abnormalities of glucose metabolism; 30–60 per cent of women with PCOS have demonstrable insulin resistance.

*See Chapter 53, Polycystic ovarian syndrome.*

## 148. PCOS is associated with:

A. Increased levels of SHBG.                                 **False**
B. Increased ovarian production of DHEAS.                    **False**
C. Increased ovarian production of androstenedione.          **True**
D. Increased ovarian production of testosterone.             **True**
E. Unopposed oestrogenic stimulation of the endometrium.     **True**

Polycystic ovarian syndrome is associated with several abnormalities of steroid metabolism. There are decreased levels of SHBG in women with PCOS. This, in combination with the increased production of adrenal DHEAS, causes an excess of free circulating androgens. The ovary also increases its production of androgens, with increases in both testosterone and androstenedione. In the long term, anovulation leads to unopposed oestrogenic stimulation of the endometrium.

*See Chapter 53, Polycystic ovarian syndrome.*

**149. With respect to androgen production in the female:**

| | |
|---|---|
| A. Testosterone is the main adrenal androgen. | **False** |
| B. Androstenedione is the main ovarian androgen. | **False** |
| C. Androstenedione and dehydroepiandrosterone (DHEA) do not have androgenic activity. | **True** |
| D. DHEAS is almost exclusively of adrenal origin. | **True** |
| E. Androstenedione and DHEA are converted to testosterone in peripheral tissues. | **True** |

Testosterone is the major circulating androgen in females; it is produced by the ovaries and the adrenals. However, approximately 50 per cent of it comes from the peripheral conversion of other androgens, including androstenedione. Androstenedione is produced in equal amounts by both the ovary and the adrenal glands. Additional androgens, including DHEAS, are almost exclusively produced by the adrenal cortex. Androstenedione and DHEA both require conversion by the enzyme 5-alpha reductase to testosterone before they are biologically active.

*See Chapter 54, Hirsutism and virilism.*

**150. When a 30-year-old woman presents with rapidly progressive hirsutism and virilization:**

| | |
|---|---|
| A. Ovarian hilus cell tumour is a possible diagnosis. | **True** |
| B. Ovarian granulosa theca cell tumour is a likely diagnosis. | **False** |
| C. A tumour of the adrenal medulla is a possible cause. | **False** |
| D. Excision of an androgen-producing ovarian tumour results in a rapid regression of hirsutism. | **False** |
| E. PCOS is a possible diagnosis. | **False** |

The term hilus cell tumour is reserved for Leydig cell tumours that are located in the ovarian hilum. Leydig cell tumours characteristically produce testosterone, are almost invariably benign in nature and occur predominantly over the age of 50 years. Steroid-producing ovarian granulosa cell tumours classically produce oestrogen and only rarely secrete testosterone. Tumours of the adrenal cortex, such as adenomas, secrete testosterone and therefore cause virilism and hirsutism. Although PCOS causes hirsutism, it does not cause virilism.

*See Chapter 54, Hirsutism and virilism.*

### 151. The following drugs are associated with hirsutism:

| | |
|---|---|
| A. Danazol. | **True** |
| B. Phenytoin. | **True** |
| C. Cyclosporin A. | **True** |
| D. Norethisterone. | **True** |
| E. Finasteride. | **False** |

The most common side effects of danazol are weight gain, fluid retention, fatigue, decreased breast size, acne, oily skin, growth of facial hair, atrophic vaginitis, hot flushes and muscle cramps. At higher doses it also causes an irreversible deepening of the voice. Long-term therapy with phenytoin causes hirsutism, acne and red-pink discoloration of urine. Norethisterone and norgestimate are derivatives of 19-nortestosterone and are both androgenic. This androgenic effect is due to their dual pharmacological action, displacing testosterone from SHBG to increase the free testosterone and bind directly to testosterone receptors. Cyclosporin A has the recognized side effect of hirsutism. Finasteride is a 5-alpha reductase inhibitor, which, as a result of its mode of action, is significantly teratogenic (emasculation of male fetus) and therefore effective contraception must always be used.

*See Chapter 54, Hirsutism and virilism.*

### 152. With respect to drug treatment for hirsutism:

| | |
|---|---|
| A. The COCP reduces SHBG production. | **False** |
| B. Medroxyprogesterone acetate reduces LH production. | **True** |
| C. Progestogens inhibit 5-alpha reductase activity. | **False** |
| D. Flutamide is a 5-alpha reductase inhibitor. | **False** |
| E. Finasteride is a testosterone antagonist. | **False** |

The oral contraceptive will suppress ovarian androgen activity and increase SHBG, thus decreasing free testosterone. Medroxyprogesterone acetate has several independent biological functions that combine to reduce the circulating levels of testosterone. It suppresses LH and ovarian testosterone production as well as increasing the testosterone clearance rates, causing an overall reduction in the circulating levels. It does not appear to affect 5-alpha reductase activity. Flutamide and finasteride are pure non-steroidal anti-androgens. These are 5-alpha reductase inhibitors.

*See Chapter 54, Hirsutism and virilism.*

**153. The following syndromes are typically associated with primary amenorrhoea:**

| | |
|---|---|
| A. Rokitansky's syndrome. | **True** |
| B. Turner's syndrome. | **True** |
| C. Sheehan's syndrome. | **False** |
| D. Kallmann's syndrome. | **True** |
| E. Asherman's syndrome. | **False** |

Rokitansky's syndrome is the congenital absence of the uterus and upper vagina due to failure of development of the Müllerian ducts. Affected girls normally present with primary amenorrhoea, and an ultrasound scan will demonstrate the absence or rudimentary development of the uterus. Women with Turner's syndrome normally have premature ovarian failure and therefore present with primary amenorrhoea. Kallmann's syndrome is a rare autosomal dominant condition with incomplete agenesis of the olfactory bulbs together with an anatomical defect of the hypothalamus. The anatomical lesion in the hypothalamus causes the absence of luteinizing hormone-releasing hormone (LHRH), and therefore hypogonado-trophic hypogonadism. Sheenan's syndrome presents with secondary amenorrhoea as a result of hypovolaemic pituitary infarction. Asherman's syndrome is secondary amenorrhoea resulting from over-vigorous curettage of the uterus.

*See Chapter 55, Amenorrhoea and oligomenorrhoea.*

**154. The following are likely diagnoses in a 16-year-old female with primary amenorrhoea but normal development of the breasts and external genitalia.**

| | |
|---|---|
| A. Turner's syndrome. | **False** |
| B. Complete androgen insensitivity syndrome. | **True** |
| C. Uterine agenesis. | **True** |
| D. Kallmann's syndrome. | **False** |
| E. Hyperprolactinaemia. | **True** |

Turner's syndrome usually presents to the gynaecologist with primary amenorrhoea and no secondary sexual characteristics. Girls with complete androgen insensitivity usually present with primary amenorrhoea. Although they have a normal 46XY karyotype, they have normal female genitalia, although sparse pubic hair. The breasts have normal duct and glandular tissue, although the areola is often underdeveloped. Girls with uterine agenesis have absent or rudimentary uterus and vagina, but normally functioning ovaries. Hyperprolactinaemia will cause amenorrhoea at any age and therefore should always be considered as a potential cause for a primary amenorrhoea.

*See Chapter 55, Amenorrhoea and oligomenorrhoea.*

**155. Gonadectomy is indicated because of the risk of malignancy in women with primary amenorrhoea and the following conditions:**

A. Turner's syndrome.                                                      **False**
B. Androgen insensitivity syndrome.                                        **True**
C. Gonadal dysgenesis with 46XY karyotype.                                 **True**
D. Gonadal dysgenesis with 46XX karyotype.                                 **False**
E. Rokitansky's syndrome.                                                  **False**

Androgen insensitivity and gonadal dysgenesis with the presence of a Y chromosome represent syndromes in which there are intra-abdominal dysgenetic testes. If the testes are left in situ, there is a 30 per cent risk of malignant change and they should therefore be removed at a suitable point after the diagnosis is confirmed.

*See Chapter 55, Amenorrhoea and oligomenorrhoea.*

**156. The following diagnoses are likely in a 30-year-old woman with secondary amenorrhoea and low gonadotrophin levels:**

A. Premature ovarian failure.                                              **False**
B. Resistant ovary syndrome.                                               **False**
C. Sheehan's syndrome.                                                     **True**
D. Asherman's syndrome.                                                    **False**
E. Post-pill amenorrhoea.                                                  **False**

Although premature ovarian failure would present with secondary amenorrhoea, the FSH would be significantly elevated. In resistant ovarian syndrome, the ovarian follicles become temporarily resistant to the actions of gonadotrophins, therefore these would be expected to be elevated. The aetiology of this disorder is thought to be autoimmune; however, the exact pathophysiology remains to be elucidated. The syndrome is characterized by amenorrhoea and high gonadotrophin levels. Amenorrhoea secondary to Sheehan's syndrome would present with low gonadotrophin levels. Both Asherman's syndrome and post-pill amenorrhoea would have normal gonadotrophin levels.

*See Chapter 55, Amenorrhoea and oligomenorrhoea.*

### 157. Regarding the menopause:

A. In the Western world between 70 and 80 per cent of women going through the menopause experience hot flushes.    **True**

B. Most oral oestrogens lead to an increase in high-density lipoprotein (HDL) cholesterol and a fall in LDL cholesterol.    **True**

C. Women with a fractured neck of femur have a 40 per cent chance of dying within a year.    **False**

D. Alzheimer's disease accounts for more than 50 per cent of all cases of dementia.    **True**

E. All women receiving hormone replacement therapy (HRT) should have a pelvic and breast examination, their weight should be measured, and blood taken for electrolyte and lipid levels before commencing therapy.    **False**

In the Western world, 70–80 per cent of women experiencing the menopause have hot flushes and sweats, which usually continue for over a year and, in up to 25 per cent of cases, for over 5 years. Oral oestrogens cause an increase in HDL and a decrease in LDL cholesterol concentrations. This should have a beneficial effect on cardiovascular disease; however, they also elevate triglyceride levels that are associated with an increased cardiovascular disease risk. Women who fracture the neck of femur have a 25 per cent chance of dying within a year and a 50 per cent chance of not being able to resume their social independence.

Alzheimer's disease accounts for 50–65 per cent of cases of dementia. Although there are no essential investigations that must be carried out before commencing HRT, it should be regarded as a screening opportunity.

*See Chapter 56, Menopause and hormone replacement therapy.*

**158.  Regarding treatment of the menopause:**

A. Double-blind studies have shown clonidine to be effective in the treatment of hot flushes and night sweats.                                                        **False**

B. Continuous combined preparations are more effective than sequential preparations at preventing endometrial cancer.                                                        **True**

C. Progestogenic side effects include bloating, mastalgia, fluid retention and acne.    **True**

D. Fifty per cent of women discontinue HRT within 3 years of starting treatment.    **False**

E. Patients with breast cancer should never receive HRT.                            **False**

Clonidine has been suggested as a possible agent for the control of hot flushes and night sweats. However, in controlled trials it has not been demonstrated to have any beneficial effect. Evidence exists that more than 5 years' usage of sequential regimens increases the risk of endometrial carcinoma. This is not seen with combined continuous regimens and there may be a reduced risk of endometrial carcinoma. Therefore women should consider changing from a sequential regimen after a few years to continuous combined therapy for long-term therapy. Progestogens can cause many side effects, including bloating, fluid retention and mastalgia, but they can be administered vaginally as a gel or pessary, therefore reducing these troublesome effects. Several studies have demonstrated a high discontinuation rate for HRT, in the region of 50 per cent within 6 months and 75 per cent within 3 years. Although to date there are no randomized, controlled trials (RCTs) of HRT post-breast cancer, several small studies have demonstrated that there does not appear to be an increase in recurrence risk in women who are prescribed HRT. However, prescribing HRT to women with a history of breast cancer should be undertaken with caution until the evidence is stronger.

*See Chapter 56, Menopause and hormone replacement therapy.*

### 159. In the management of bleeding in early pregnancy:

A. The beta subunit of human chorionic gonadotrophin (βhCG) measured in maternal blood originates from the fetus.                                                                                      **False**

B. At 7 weeks' gestation, an observed increase of βhCG from 1500 to 2000 IU/ml over 48 hours is likely to indicate the presence of an early viable intrauterine pregnancy.                                                                                   **False**

C. An unruptured tubal ectopic pregnancy in a 22-year-old nulliparous woman with previous unilateral salpingectomy is best treated with salpingectomy.            **False**

D. Methotrexate treatment of an unruptured tubal ectopic pregnancy results in a prompt fall in concentrations of βhCG measured in maternal blood.                    **False**

E. In the days following methotrexate treatment, patients should be advised to avoid the use of non-steroidal anti-inflammatory drugs (NSAIDs).                            **True**

The βhCG measured in maternal blood originates in the placenta, not the developing fetus. The modern radioimmunoassay for βhCG detects levels at 5 IU/L. Therefore, increases in βhCG are first seen in the serum at 9 days and in the urine at 13 days following ovulation. During early pregnancy, the βhCG should double over a 48-hour period, and anything less should alert the clinician to the possibility of an ectopic pregnancy. An unruptured tubal pregnancy in a 22-year-old woman who is known to have had a salpingectomy should be treated as conservatively as possible to allow possible further pregnancies. Treatment would depend on whether the ectopic pregnancy fulfilled the criteria for conservative management, medical management or required surgical intervention. The treatment of an ectopic pregnancy with methotrexate initially causes the βhCG levels to rise, but by day 7 they should be at least 15 per cent less than the pre-treatment level and should fall substantially each week after that. Monitoring should continue until the βhCG is <25 IU/L, which can take up to 4 weeks.

Non-steroidal anti-inflammatory drugs decrease renal elimination of methotrexate and also displace it from plasma protein binding sites, thus enhancing their toxicity. Omeprazole, high-dose penicillins and sulphonamides also increase toxicity. Alcohol enhances the hepatotoxicity. Broad-spectrum antibiotics should be avoided, as they decrease methotrexate serum levels and efficacy after oral administration.

*See Chapter 57, Problems in early pregnancy.*

**160.  Following complete miscarriage of a first pregnancy at 6 weeks' gestation:**

A. Attempts to conceive again should be avoided for three menstrual cycles.    **False**

B. Failure to give anti-D to Rhesus (Rh)-negative patients is likely to lead to Rh sensitization in a subsequent pregnancy.    **False**

C. The risk of miscarriage of the second pregnancy is approximately 25 per cent.    **False**

D. Diagnosis should be confirmed by dilatation and curettage.    **False**

E. The couple should be offered a thrombophilia screen.    **False**

There is no evidence to suggest that a couple should avoid attempts to conceive for three cycles; it should be when the couple feels that it is most appropriate to try. The RCOG guideline on anti-D prophylaxis suggests that anti-D does not need to be administered until after 10 weeks, or if the patient requires a surgical intervention. A thrombophilia screen should only be offered after three recurrent spontaneous miscarriages with the same partner. Dilatation and curettage is not required following a complete miscarriage.

*See Chapter 57, Problems in early pregnancy.*

**161.  With regard to urinary tract infections (UTIs):**

A. Overall, 5 per cent of women have asymptomatic bacteriuria.    **True**

B. Thirty per cent of women will develop a UTI in their lifetime.    **False**

C. *Escherichia coli* is the main causative organism.    **True**

D. Recurrent UTIs are rarely caused by the same organism.    **False**

E. Urethral catheters are associated with higher rates of infection than suprapubic catheters.    **True**

Lower urinary tract infection is common; 5 per cent of women have been found to have asymptomatic bacteriuria and 50 per cent of women will experience a UTI in their lifetime. *Escherichia coli* is the most commonly isolated organism, and recurrent lower UTIs tend to be associated with the same infective organism. Suprapubic catheters are preferred to urethral catheters for long-term catheterization, as they are associated with a lower incidence of infection.

*See Chapter 61, Lower urinary tract infections.*

### 162. Considering the treatment of urinary tract infections:

| | |
|---|---|
| A. Bacteriuria should usually be treated. | **False** |
| B. Bacteriuria should usually be treated in pregnancy. | **True** |
| C. Cranberry juice has been proven to be effective. | **True** |
| D. Amoxycillin is effective as a single-dose agent. | **False** |
| E. Vaginal oestrogens are effective in the management of postmenopausal women with recurrent UTIs. | **True** |

Asymptomatic bacteriuria does not always warrant treatment, although it should be treated in pregnancy as it may be associated with preterm delivery. Cranberry juice has been shown to offer effective prophylaxis by preventing colonization of the lower urinary tract; by lowering the vaginal pH, topical vaginal oestrogens are effective in postmenopausal women. Many different antibiotic regimens are commonly used, although amoxycillin has not been shown to be effective as a single-dose agent.

*See Chapter 61, Lower urinary tract infections.*

### 163. Urogenital prolapse:

| | |
|---|---|
| A. Accounts for 50 per cent of all gynaecological procedures. | **False** |
| B. Rarely occurs in nulliparous women. | **True** |
| C. May be associated with lower urinary tract symptoms. | **True** |
| D. Is more common following the menopause. | **True** |
| E. Is found in 30 per cent of elderly women. | **False** |

Urogenital prolapse is a common gynaecological condition, accounting for 20 per cent of major gynaecological procedures, rising to 59 per cent of procedures in the elderly. Although more common in women who have had children, it may also occur in nulliparous women and may be associated with connective tissue disease.

Urogenital prolapse is often associated with concomitant lower urinary tract symptoms such as stress or urge incontinence and is more common following the withdrawal of endogenous oestrogens at the menopause, affecting a third of elderly women.

*See Chapter 62, Urogenital prolapse.*

## 164. With regard to the management of urogenital prolapse:

| | |
|---|---|
| A. Physiotherapy has been shown to be effective. | **False** |
| B. Ring pessaries are the management of choice in the elderly. | **False** |
| C. Sacrospinous ligament fixation should be performed routinely at vaginal hysterectomy to prevent vault prolapse. | **False** |
| D. Enterocele formation is increased following colposuspension. | **True** |
| E. Anterior repair is an effective treatment for co-existent stress incontinence. | **False** |

Whereas physiotherapy has been shown to be effective in the management of women complaining of stress incontinence, this is not the case when considering prolapse. Surgery remains the management of choice, and ring pessaries should only be considered for those women who decline surgery, wish to have more children or are medically unfit. Sacrospinous ligament fixation may be offered to women complaining of vaginal vault prolapse, although it should not be performed routinely at the time of vaginal hysterectomy, as it alters the axis of the vagina and may lead to urinary symptoms and dyspareunia. Equally, correction of the anterior wall prolapse at the time of colposuspension may predispose to posterior compartment defects such as rectocele or enterocele. Anterior repair, with a success rate of approximately 60 per cent at 2-year follow-up, should no longer be considered as a treatment for urodynamic stress incontinence.

*See Chapter 62, Urogenital prolapse.*

## 165. The following investigations are useful in women suspected of having PID:

| | |
|---|---|
| A. Pregnancy test. | **True** |
| B. Endocervical test for *Chlamydia trachomatis*. | **True** |
| C. Endocervical test for *Neisseria gonorrhoeae*. | **True** |
| D. Erythrocyte sedimentation rate (ESR). | **True** |
| E. Carcinoembryonic antigen (CEA). | **False** |
| F. Plain abdominal X-ray. | **False** |

It is imperative to exclude ectopic pregnancy in this group. Chlamydial and gonococcal infections are well-described, important causes of PID. The ESR can be raised in PID, as can the C-reactive protein (CRP). Carcinoembryonic antigen is a tumour marker and has not been used in the investigation of PID. Ultrasound of the pelvis is occasionally useful as a diagnostic tool, but plain X-rays are not used in this situation.

*See Chapter 63.1, Infection and sexual health.*

### 166. The following are signs and symptoms of PID:

A. Lower abdominal pain.                                    **True**

B. Dyspareunia.                                            **True**

C. Menorrhagia as a new symptom.                          **True**

D. Abnormal vaginal discharge.                            **True**

E. Cervical excitation.                                   **True**

F. Right upper quadrant discomfort.                       **True**

G. Breakthrough bleeding on the COCP.                     **True**

Any unscheduled bleeding can be a sign of endometritis, due to pelvic infection. Right upper quadrant discomfort may be a sign of perihepatitis, due to ascending infection to the liver capsule in PID.

*See Chapter 63.1, Infection and sexual health.*

### 167. *Chlamydia trachomatis*:

A. Is diagnosed by culture of cervical purulent discharge.                    **False**

B. Has been found to be carried by an increased number of women using the COCP.   **True**

C. Is usually symptomatic.                                                     **False**

D. Is routinely treated with penicillins.                                      **False**

*Chlamydia trachomatis* is isolated by various techniques using endocervical cells and not pus. The infection is asymptomatic in 80 per cent of women and in 50 per cent of men. It is routinely treated with tetracyclines, except in pregnancy, when macrolides are generally used.

*See Chapter 63.1, Infection and sexual health.*

### 168. With regard to genital herpes simplex infection in pregnancy:

A. Aciclovir is not used.                                                       **False**

B. Vaginal delivery would be anticipated except for those developing symptoms of a first episode after 34 weeks' gestation.                              **True**

C. Continuous antiviral therapy is indicated in the last 4 weeks of pregnancy in those who have a first episode of infection in the first and second trimesters of pregnancy.                                                         **True**

D. It is diagnosed by high vaginal swab.                                        **False**

Aciclovir is not licensed for use in pregnancy, but there is enough clinical evidence supporting its safety. Caesarean section should be considered for those developing symptoms of a first episode of genital herpes simplex infection after 34 weeks, as the risk of viral shedding in labour is very high. For those who develop a first episode in the first and second trimesters, vaginal delivery would be anticipated; continuous aciclovir in the last 4 weeks reduces the risk of recurrence at term and caesarean section.

*See Chapter 63.1, Infection and sexual health.*

### 169. Dyspareunia is associated with:

A. Vaginal infection.                                            **True**

B. Allergic dermatitis of the vulva.                            **True**

C. Involuntary spasm of the pubo-coccygeal muscles.             **True**

D. Poor sexual technique.                                        **True**

E. UTI.                                                          **True**

Any infection or underlying skin problem of the vulva and vagina can cause painful intercourse (dyspareunia). Vaginismus is involuntary spasm of the pelvic floor muscles and can cause dyspareunia. Inadequate sexual stimulation can cause lack of vaginal lubrication and therefore dyspareunia.

*See Chapter 63.2, Dyspareunia and other psychosexual problems.*

### 170. With regard to sexual history taking:

A. Gynaecologists do not need to be comfortable to talk about sexual intercourse in
   detail.                                                       **False**

B. The age of the adult patient should determine whether sex is mentioned during
   the consultation.                                             **False**

C. Talking about sex prior to gynaecological surgery is not appropriate.   **False**

Talking about sex with patients should take place during gynaecological history taking for all adults and gynaecologists should feel comfortable to do so. 'Is sex comfortable for you?' or 'Are there any problems with sex?' is all that is required to enable the patient to raise issues pertaining to sexual problems. It is important to establish issues to do with sex prior to surgery, in case they affect the patient's management.

*See Chapter 63.2, Dyspareunia and other psychosexual problems.*

### 171. Child sex abuse:

A. Cannot take place in children under 3 years of age.          **False**

B. Includes exposure.                                            **True**

C. Can be managed solely by the gynaecologist who diagnoses the problem.   **False**

D. Can be diagnosed confidently after discovering that a 13-year-old is not virgo
   intacta.                                                      **False**

Child sex abuse can take place at any age under 18 years. Exposure is the viewing of sexual acts, pornography and exhibitionism and is considered as part of the spectrum of child sex abuse. Gynaecologists must involve a designated paediatrician as soon as they have any suspicion. Thirteen-year-old girls may have been having consensual sex. It is important to establish the nature of the relationship in all sexually active under-16 year olds in order to exclude child sex abuse.

*See Chapter 63.3, Child sex abuse.*

**172. The following may be adult sequelae of child sex abuse:**

A. Persistent vaginal discharge.                                    **True**

B. Anxiety disorders.                                               **True**

C. Promiscuity.                                                     **True**

D. Alcohol abuse.                                                   **True**

Patients may present in a variety of ways to a variety of healthcare professionals. A variety of gynaecological disorders may present as a sequel to child sex abuse, e.g. vaginal discharge, pelvic pain.

*See Chapter 63.3, Child sex abuse.*

**173. With regard to the management of rape victims:**

A. The timing of the examination is not relevant.                  **False**

B. Forensic sampling is the priority of the examination.           **False**

C. Informed consent should be obtained prior to the forensic medical examination.   **True**

D. Clothing should not be sent for forensic examination.           **False**

E. Screening for sexually transmitted diseases should be offered to the victim.   **True**

The examination of an alleged rape victim should take place as soon as possible after the assault. The management of injuries requiring urgent medical attention takes priority over the forensic medical examination. Consent must be obtained for a medical examination (non-genital and genital), the collection of forensic evidence, the retention of relevant items of clothing for forensic examination, and the disclosure of details of medical record to the police and/or Crown Prosecution Service (CPS). Clothing should be sent for forensic examination, provided consent has been obtained. All rape victims should be offered screening for sexually transmitted diseases, including HIV disease.

*See Chapter 63.4, Rape and rape counselling.*

**174. With regard to rape:**

A. It is defined as 'unlawful sexual intercourse by a woman with a man, by force, fear or fraud'.   **False**

B. Rape victims should be examined by specialist forensic medical examiners.   **True**

C. Fifty per cent of rape victims have major non-genital injuries.   **False**

D. Genital photographs should be taken by a photographer of a different gender.   **False**

E. Post-exposure HIV prophylaxis should be continued for 3 months.   **False**

Rape is defined as 'unlawful sexual intercourse by a man with a woman, by force, fear or fraud' (Sexual Offences Act 1956, England). All victims of sexual assault should be examined by forensic medical examiners who have received specific training in forensic gynaecology (police surgeons). Up to 5 per cent of rape victims have major non-genital injuries.

Any genital or intimate photographs must be taken by a photographer of the same gender.

Post-exposure HIV prophylaxis with zidovudine and lamivudine plus nelfinavir or indinavir should be continued for 28 days and involves a negative baseline HIV ELISA test, pre-HIV test counselling, informed consent and monitoring by an HIV specialist.

*See Chapter 63.4, Rape and rape counselling.*

**175.  With regard to vulval lichen sclerosus:**

A. Histological diagnosis is mandatory.                                     **False**

B. Emollient creams are ineffective.                                        **False**

C. Eighty per cent of cases will respond to 1% hydrocortisone cream.        **False**

D. Testosterone cream is useful for maintaining response.                   **False**

E. The condition is usually self-limiting.                                  **False**

The history and clinical characteristics of lichen sclerosus are usually obvious and biopsy would only be considered mandatory if there were features suspicious of malignancy or there had not been the expected response to topical steroids and emollients. Emollients should always be considered in treatment, particularly when a response has been achieved with steroids and a long-term maintenance therapy is required.

Topical fluorinated steroids are the mainstay of primary therapy. Long-term use of these preparations may be associated with toxicity and, if possible, the dose should be reduced or emollients used instead. Weaker steroids such as 1% hydrocortisone are not very effective in bringing about remission.

Testosterone cream has been used, but there is no objective evidence that it is of any value in either inducing a remission or maintaining it. Maintaining remissions is important in this condition, which is virtually always chronic with exacerbation. It is not self-limiting, and this fact is an important one to convey to women who have the condition.

*See Chapter 64, Benign vulval problems.*

**176.  With regard to vulval skin diseases:**

A. Seborrhoeic dermatitis is a fungal condition.                            **True**

B. Hidradenitis suppurativa is a disorder of the eccrine glands.            **False**

C. Psoriasis affecting the vulva is best managed with tar preparations.     **False**

D. In vulvovaginal candidiasis, topical antifungals are less effective than oral
   preparations.                                                            **False**

E. Lichen planus is a pre-malignant condition.                              **True**

*Malassemia ovalis* is a yeast that plays a central role in the pathogenesis of seborrhoeic dermatitis; the primary choice of treatment is an antifungal preparation.

Hidradenitis suppurativa is a chronic, suppurative, inflammatory disorder of the apocrine glands. It is characterized by deep, painful, subcutaneous nodules that may ulcerate and drain, leading to open sinuses and extensive scarring. On the vulva, the disease primarily affects the labia majora and intercrural folds, but may also involve the mons pubis, labia minora and clitoris.

With regard to the treatment of psoriasis, emollients and keratolytics have no proven benefit and tar preparations should be avoided, as they are irritating.

In psoriasis in general, topical steroids are beneficial in the short term, but prolonged use should be avoided. Vitamin D derivatives may be as effective as steroids, but without the risk of skin atrophy, although irritation may be a problem.

No differences exist in terms of the relative effectiveness of antifungals administered by the oral or intravaginal routes for the treatment of uncomplicated vaginal candidiasis.

*See Chapter 64, Benign vulval problems.*

### 177. In vulval vestibulitis:

A. Pain is occasionally associated with light touch in the vestibule area.                  **False**

B. Vestibular erythema is necessary to make a diagnosis.                  **False**

C. The modified vestibulectomy produces a success rate of 70 per cent in well-selected patients.                  **True**

D. Sensate focus therapy should complement the physical treatments among those patients with sexual dysfunction.                  **True**

E. Amitryptyline is the first-line treatment of choice.                  **False**

Vestibular hyperaesthesia is essential to make a diagnosis, and vestibular erythema is common and seen in asymptomatic women. Several reported series have indicated success varying between 60 and 80 per cent with the modified vestibulectomy procedure. These patients have to be carefully selected. In those women in whom secondary psychosexual problems have arisen as a result of pain during intercourse, appropriate psychosexual therapy should be considered.

Amitryptyline is useful for the neuropathic pain of dysaesthetic vulvodynia, but not usually for vulval vestibulitis.

*See Chapter 65, Vulval pain syndromes.*

### 178. In dysaesthetic vulvodynia:

A. The pain experienced by the patient is typically neuropathic.                  **True**

B. Patients are usually 20–30 years of age.                  **False**

C. The standard dosage of amitryptyline is 10 mg/day.                  **False**

D. Irritant contact dermatitis of the vulva can occur.                  **True**

E. Peri-anal pain may also occur.                  **True**

Neuropathic pain is the classical pain type seen in dysaesthetic vulvodynia. This is burning and/or lancinating in character. Patients are usually 40–60 years old.

Amitryptyline is usually the first choice and doses of up to 60 mg/day are regarded as standard. The vulval epithelium is usually normal on inspection, with none of the features associated with an irritative dermatitis.

There is an overlap with pudendal neuralgia resulting in perineal pain of a similar nature.

*See Chapter 65, Vulval pain syndromes.*

## 179.  With regard to human papillomaviruses (HPVs):

A. They are RNA viruses of about 8000 base pairs.                           **False**

B. HPV 16 is the commonest oncogenic genital type.                          **True**

C. Different types can be distinguished by electron microscopy.             **False**

D. The prevalence of genital HPV infection decreases with advancing age.    **True**

E. The host's main response to infection is antibody mediated.              **False**

Human papillomaviruses are DNA viruses with a circular or superhelical form for the 7900 base pairs. The most common oncogenic subtype is HPV 16. It is impossible to differentiate HPV types by their electron microscopic appearance; this is determined by characterizing their genomic organization.

Infection appears to be far more prevalent in the early reproductive years and this may reflect developing natural immunity and the ability to eliminate virus and prevent re-infection in later years. The main host response to HPV infection is cell mediated.

*See Chapter 66, Pre-invasive disease.*

## 180.  With regard to the National Health Service (NHS) cervical screening
##        programme:

A. Since organized screening was introduced, there has been a fall in the incidence of
   cervical cancer.                                                         **True**

B. More than 80 per cent of eligible women are covered by the programme.    **True**

C. About 25 per cent of smears are reported as 'not normal'.                **False**

D. Women are screened with a maximum 3-yearly cycle.                        **False**

E. General practitioners are paid according to whether they meet coverage targets for
   cervical smears.                                                         **True**

The most significant fall in the incidence of cervical cancer in the UK occurred following the introduction of an organized screening programme. Nationally, this has now achieved in excess of 80 per cent coverage of the eligible population; one of the important reasons for this has been incentive payments to primary care to encourage the achievement of targets.

Screening begins between the ages of 20 and 25 years and continues to the age of 65 years. The interval between tests should not exceed 5 years, although some health authorities offer screening on a 3-yearly basis. About 10 per cent of all screening smears are 'not normal', although the majority of the non-negative smears are either minor abnormalities or inadequate specimens.

*See Chapter 66, Pre-invasive disease.*

### 181. In the investigation of postmenopausal bleeding:

A. TVUS has a high sensitivity.                                    **True**

B. Magnetic resonance imaging (MRI) should be used if available.    **False**

C. Endometrial biopsy is often necessary.                          **False**

D. Outpatient hysteroscopy is the investigation of choice.         **False**

E. Pelvic examination can be replaced by TVUS.                     **False**

Transvaginal ultrasound as a modality for assessing postmenopausal bleeding has a sensitivity of 94–100 per cent for the detection of endometrial pathology. The variation in the sensitivity depends on the cut-off point used for endometrial thickness. The negative predictive value of TVUS is 100 per cent, therefore a normal value needs no further investigation. Both MRI scans and ultrasound can be used for the staging of endometrial cancer; however, the role of MRI is still unclear. At the present time, MRI has no role in the investigation of postmenopausal bleeding. As an initial investigation of postmenopausal bleeding, outpatient hysteroscopy is considered to be too invasive. This is particularly the case when one considers the sensitivity and specificity of ultrasound.

*See Chapter 67, Endometrial cancer.*

### 182. Following surgery for endometrial cancer:

A. Vault brachytherapy will improve survival.                      **False**

B. HRT is contraindicated.                                         **False**

C. Pelvic irradiation will reduce the risk of pelvic recurrence.   **True**

D. Tamoxifen for a previous breast cancer may be continued.        **True**

E. Adjuvant progesterone therapy is not usually of benefit.        **True**

Although vault radiotherapy has been shown to reduce local and regional recurrences, none of the studies performed has shown any effect on survival rates. Most endometrial cancers are oestrogen responsive and therefore traditionally HRT has been avoided. However, recent data suggest that there is no reduction in the recurrence interval with the use of HRT, and therefore it should not be withheld if there is a clinical indication. Adjuvant progesterone therapy for early-stage disease has not been shown to improve overall survival and therefore its use cannot be advocated.

*See Chapter 67, Endometrial cancer.*

### 183. With regard to micro-invasive disease:

A. It is associated with nodal disease in 20 per cent of cases.                     **False**
B. It can be cured by large loop excision of the transformation zone (LLETZ).       **True**
C. It is associated with a depth of invasion of 9 mm.                               **False**
D. It always requires radical hysterectomy.                                         **False**
E. Pelvic lymphadenectomy should only be performed in selected cases.               **True**

Micro-invasive disease of the cervix comprises 20 per cent of the cervical cancers and is subclassified according to the depth of stromal invasion. Stromal invasion of <3 mm is stage Ia1 disease and associated with <1 per cent lymph node involvement. Therefore, if a LLETZ has adequate resection margins and the invasion of the stroma is <3 mm, no further treatment is required. Stromal invasion of between 3 mm and 5 mm is stage Ia2 and is associated with lymph node involvement of approximately 5 per cent. Therefore, lymph node dissection should be considered for this group of patients, but the decision should be based on lymph/vascular space involvement.

*See Chapter 68, Cervical cancer.*

### 184. With regard to stage Ib cervical cancer:

A. Squamous carcinoma is the most common type.                                      **True**
B. Small-cell type is associated with distant metastases.                           **True**
C. It can be treated by chemoradiotherapy.                                          **True**
D. Following surgery, disease-free vaginal margins of <5 mm should be considered for
   adjuvant chemotherapy.                                                           **True**
E. Radical surgery is associated with chronic voiding problems.                     **True**

Squamous cell carcinoma of the cervix constitutes 85 per cent of cervical cancer. Small-cell cancer of the cervix is characteristically associated with a later presentation and early distant metastasis. Several recent trials have demonstrated a significant survival advantage to women given cisplatin-based therapy concurrently with radiation therapy. Women with resected positive pelvic nodes should be offered adjuvant radiotherapy to reduce the risk of recurrence. However, patients with vaginal margins of <0.5 cm may also benefit from pelvic irradiation. Radical hysterectomy is associated with a number of postoperative problems, which include chronic bladder and bowel dysfunction.

*See Chapter 68, Cervical cancer.*

### 185. In the treatment of ovarian cancer:

A. Standard adjuvant therapy involves intravenous chemotherapy. **True**

B. Adjuvant therapy is not indicated for patients with stage Ic disease. **False**

C. Paclitaxel and carboplatin are prescribed for patients with advanced disease. **True**

D. Alkylating agents are the mainstay of treatment. **False**

E. Response rates to second-line chemotherapy are of the order of 70 per cent. **False**

All the standard chemotherapy regimens in the UK involve intravenous administration. Adjuvant chemotherapy is not indicated in low-grade stage Ia or b disease. However, patients with high-grade disease or greater than stage Ib disease have been demonstrated to have a survival advantage and a longer disease-free interval with adjuvant chemotherapy. Paclitaxel and carboplatin are used in the treatment of advanced ovarian cancer. Although alone they have both been shown to improve survival, there effectiveness in combination is less clear-cut. The response of ovarian cancer to second-line treatment is in the region of 15–35 per cent, compared with an 80 per cent response to primary chemotherapy.

*See Chapter 69, Benign and malignant ovarian masses.*

### 186. Malignant germ-cell tumours:

A. Account for 15 per cent of all ovarian malignances. **False**

B. Represent 60 per cent of ovarian cancers in children and adolescents. **True**

C. Are usually bilateral. **False**

D. Have an overall 5-year survival rate of 38 per cent. **False**

E. Require treatment that usually results in infertility. **False**

Approximately 30 per cent of benign and malignant ovarian tumours are of germ-cell origin. Although only a small proportion of these will be malignant, they do represent 60 per cent of ovarian cancers in the first two decades of life. The two most common histological types of germ-cell tumour are the dysgerminoma and the immature teratoma. However, unlike other malignant tumours of the ovary, the majority are unilateral in nature. The standard management of these tumours is conservative, with removal of the affected ovary in combination with chemotherapy; this is curative in most cases. Most patients who have been cured by this treatment can expect normal menstrual and reproductive function.

*See Chapter 69, Benign and malignant ovarian masses.*

**187.  With regard to cancer of the vulva:**

A. It is linked to HPV in 90 per cent of all cases.                                    **False**

B. It develops in 4 per cent of cases of lichen sclerosus.                             **True**

C. It develops in 80 per cent of cases of treated vulval intraepithelial neoplasia 3
(VIN3).                                                                                **False**

D. Melanoma of the vulva is the second most common type.                               **True**

E. It most commonly affects the perineum.                                              **False**

Approximately one-third of vulval cancers can be related to oncogenic HPVs and a further third appear to be related to a pre-existing maturation disorder. The aetiology of the remainder is uncertain. The lifetime risk of developing vulval cancer with lichen sclerosus has been estimated at 4 per cent. There has been one report documenting seven out of eight cases of untreated VIN progressing to cancer. Overall, however, particularly in treated cases, the risk is probably in the order of 5–10 per cent. After squamous cancer, the next most common histological type is malignant melanoma, which accounts for less than 10 per cent of all cases.

The labia are the most frequently affected sites for malignant neoplasms.

*See Chapter 70, Vulval and vaginal cancer.*

**188.  In the treatment of vulval cancer:**

A. All stage I vulval cancers require a bilateral inguinal lymph node dissection.      **False**

B. Superficial inguinal node dissection has the same rate of groin recurrence as an
inguino-femoral node dissection.                                                       **False**

C. The risk of recurrence following surgery for stage I/II disease is the same for a
triple incision technique and an 'en-bloc' radical vulvectomy.                         **True**

D. Adjuvant radiotherapy is recommended when there is extracapsular lymph node
spread in a single lymph node.                                                         **True**

E. Chemoradiotherapy has a cure rate equivalent to that of surgery in the treatment
of stage II vulva cancer.                                                              **False**

All squamous cancers other than stage Ia carry a risk of groin node metastases in excess of 5 per cent. These require either bilateral or ipsilateral (for small lateralized tumours) lymphadenectomy. If dissection omits the deep femoral nodes, there is an increased risk of recurrence in the groin; for this reason superficial inguinal lymphadenectomy is not recommended. There is no evidence that radical en-bloc dissection is significantly better in terms of local recurrence than the more recently employed triple incision procedure. Postoperative adjuvant radiotherapy is given to the groins if there are two or more nodes with microscopic involvement or one node that is totally replaced by tumour or that demonstrates capsular breach. There are insufficient data regarding the use of chemoradiation in early vulval cancer to determine whether or not it is superior to the traditional surgical approach.

*See Chapter 70, Vulval and vaginal cancer.*

### 189. Complete hydatidiform moles:

| | |
|---|---|
| A. Are usually diploid. | **True** |
| B. Give rise to persistent trophoblastic disease in 50 per cent of cases. | **False** |
| C. Can co-exist with a normal 'twin' conceptus. | **True** |
| D. Usually present after the 16th week of pregnancy. | **False** |
| E. Are commonly repetitive. | **False** |

Complete hydatidiform moles are diploid and acquire their entire chromosomal component from the male (dispermy). About 15–20 per cent of complete moles will ultimately require chemotherapy, and it has been estimated that 3 per cent of complete moles will develop into choriocarcinoma. Twin pregnancy can occur, although the frequency is lower than in non-molar pregnancies. The majority of cases are diagnosed prior to 16 weeks' gestation with the more frequent use of early ultrasound examination. Although the risk of subsequent molar pregnancy is increased (incidence rises to 1:76 with one previous mole and 1:6.5 with two), the likelihood is that a subsequent pregnancy will not be a repeat molar pregnancy.

*See Chapter 71, Gestational trophoblastic disease.*

### 190. Partial hydatidiform moles:

| | |
|---|---|
| A. Are usually triploid. | **True** |
| B. Rarely give rise to persistent trophoblastic disease. | **True** |
| C. Often present as a missed miscarriage. | **True** |
| D. Are easy to diagnose on ultrasound scan. | **False** |
| E. Often have recognizable embryonic and fetal tissues. | **True** |

Partial hydatidiform moles are usually triploid, and fetal parts may be identifiable. They infrequently result in persistent trophoblastic disease (0.5–1 per cent). The usual presentation is that of a missed miscarriage and they usually present somewhat later than complete moles. Diagnosis on ultrasound can be difficult because of the associated fetal parts, although placental abnormalities may indicate the underlying pathology.

*See Chapter 71, Gestational trophoblastic disease.*

# Short Answer Questions

# OBSTETRICS

1. A 32-year-old multiparous women presents at 10 weeks' gestation to the antenatal clinic. She has a blood pressure of 140/90 mmHg. Outline the management of this problem.
   *See Chapter 6.1, Chronic hypertension.*

2. Evaluate the methods of fetal assessment in a woman with insulin-dependent diabetes mellitus diagnosed 3 years before conception.
   *See Chapter 6.2, Diabetes mellitus.*

3. A 24-year-old woman with poorly controlled insulin-dependent diabetes attends a pre-pregnancy clinic. Justify the advice specific to her condition that you would give.
   *See Chapter 6.2, Diabetes mellitus.*

4. A 26-year-old Asian woman attends an antenatal booking clinic. In the referral letter it is highlighted that she has an atrial septal heart lesion. Outline the subsequent management.
   *See Chapter 6.3, Cardiac disease.*

5. Discuss the management of a 34-year-old woman with a known history of Graves' disease who is contemplating pregnancy.
   *See Chapter 6.4, Thyroid disease.*

6. A 25-year-old nulliparous woman has a repeat full blood count at 28 weeks' gestation confirming a platelet count of $65 \times 10^9$/L. Outline your differential diagnosis and antenatal management.
   *See Chapter 6.5, Haematological conditions.*

7. Pulmonary embolism remains a major cause of maternal death. Outline the steps that should be taken to minimize the risk of thromboembolism in pregnant women.
   *See Chapter 6.5, Haematological conditions, and Chapter 9, Maternal mortality.*

8. A 34-year-old woman with polycystic kidneys seeks your advice as she wishes to become pregnant. Routine blood tests demonstrate that she has serum creatinine of 175 μmol/L. How would you advise her with regard to pregnancy?
   *See Chapter 6.6, Renal disease.*

9. A 37-year-old woman who is known to have systemic lupus erythematosus presents at the antenatal clinic. Outline the management of this pregnancy.
   *See Chapter 6.7, Autoimmune conditions.*

10. A 24-year-old primiparous woman presents to the accident and emergency department with persistent vomiting when 7 weeks pregnant. Outline the management of this woman.
    *See Chapter 6.8, Liver and gastrointestinal disease.*

11. A 26-year-old woman who is 36 weeks pregnant in her first pregnancy presents to the antenatal clinic with a skin rash. Briefly outline the possible differential diagnoses and how these conditions could be treated.
    *See Chapter 6.11, Dermatological conditions.*

12. A 22-year-old ex-intravenous drug abuser (currently on methadone) books at 15 weeks in her first pregnancy. She is hepatitis B positive. Outline a comprehensive plan for her care.
    *See Chapter 6.12, Drug and alcohol misuse, and Chapter 7.4, Infection.*

13. Justify the statement 'all women who smoke and are pregnant should be offered a programme for cessation of smoking'.
    *See Chapter 6.13, Smoking.*

14. A 25-year-old woman in her fourth pregnancy is seen in the booking clinic at 20 weeks' gestation. Her community midwife has taken routine bloods. Her haemoglobin concentration is 7.2 g/dL. How would you manage her pregnancy?
    *See Chapter 7.1, Anaemia.*

15. Justify the investigation of a 39-year-old woman presenting at 34 weeks' gestation with right hypochondrial pain.
    *See Chapter 7.2, Abdominal pain.*

16. A 36-year-old woman who is in her third pregnancy is referred at 30 weeks' gestation with a lump in her breast. Outline the initial investigation of this patient.
    *See Chapter 7.3, Malignancy.*

17. A 24-year-old woman in her first pregnancy is noted to have a 6 cm adnexal mass on a dating ultrasound scan at 8 weeks' gestation. Justify your management.
    *See Chapter 7.3, Malignancy.*

18. Justify the initiation of insulin therapy in a 26-year-old woman with gestational diabetes diagnosed at 20 weeks' gestation.
    *See Chapter 7.5, Gestational diabetes.*

19. A 34-year-old woman presents at 36 weeks in her second pregnancy. Her first pregnancy was complicated by an elective caesarean section for breech presentation. She has a blood pressure of 140/90 mmHg and urine Dipstix shows 2+ proteinuria. Outline the management of this woman for the rest of her pregnancy.

    *See Chapter 7.6, Pre-eclampsia and non-proteinuric pregnancy-induced hypertension, and Chapter 26, Management after previous caesarean section.*

20. Illustrate, using examples of medications prescribed for respiratory and neurological disease, how drugs and pregnancy may influence one another.

    *See Chapter 8, Medication in pregnancy.*

21. Debate the use of nuchal translucency screening versus serum screening as methods of identifying pregnancies at risk of Down's syndrome.

    *See Chapter 10.1, Biochemical screening.*

22. Discuss the aims of the mid-trimester anomaly ultrasound scan, using examples of neural tube, abdominal wall and renal abnormalities.

    *See Chapter 10.2, Ultrasound screening.*

23. Discuss the indications and drawbacks of the different methods of invasive fetal testing.

    *See Chapter 10.3, Invasive prenatal diagnosis.*

24. Discuss the management of a woman whose fetus is noted to have an abdominal wall defect when scanned at 20 weeks' gestation.

    *See Chapter 10.4, Management of fetal anomalies.*

25. Discuss the management of a 27-year-old woman who presents at an antenatal booking clinic having had a stillbirth at 27 weeks' gestation in her last pregnancy.

    *See Chapter 11, Previous history of fetal loss.*

26. Discuss the prognosis and management of a twin pregnancy complicated by fetal demise.

    *See Chapter 12, Multiple pregnancy.*

27. Describe the management of a pregnancy in which the mother has had a viral illness and has been demonstrated to have an acute cytomegalovirus infection.

    *See Chapter 13, Fetal infections.*

28. Describe the management of a pregnancy at 28 weeks' gestation where the symphysio-fundal height measures 24 cm.

    *See Chapter 14, Tests of fetal well-being, and Chapter 15, Fetal growth restriction.*

29. Describe the management of a fetus that had a 20-week scan and that has been identified as having hydrops fetalis.

    *See Chapter 17, Fetal hydrops.*

30. Discuss how you would manage a woman who is in her first pregnancy at 41 weeks' gestation and who has declined vaginal examination and induction of labour.

    *See Chapter 19, Prolonged pregnancy.*

31. A woman presents at 26 weeks with ruptured membranes. She is not contracting. Describe your management.
    *See Chapter 22, Pre-labour rupture of membranes.*

32. A 30-year-old primigravida attends the antenatal clinic 3 days after her expected date of delivery. The pregnancy has been problem free. How would you advise this woman?
    *See Chapter 25, Induction of labour.*

33. Critically comment on the management of slow progress during the active phase of the first stage of spontaneous labour in a multiparous woman.
    *See Chapter 27, Poor progress in labour.*

34. You are called to a fetal bradycardia that has occurred 10 minutes after the siting of an epidural. Discuss your management.
    *See Chapter 29, Fetal compromise in the first stage of labour.*

35. What precautions should be taken at a caesarean section for a placenta praevia in order to minimize maternal blood loss? If excess blood loss occurred, what would your management plan be?
    *See Chapter 31, Caesarean section.*

36. You are asked to assess an abnormal cardiotocogram in a woman at term in her first pregnancy. The cervix is fully dilated, but she has an effective epidural and is not pushing. Describe your management.
    *See Chapter 32, Fetal compromise in the second stage of labour.*

37. Shoulder dystocia presents a significant risk-management problem. Outline the strategies that can be employed to minimize this risk.
    *See Chapter 33, Shoulder dystocia.*

38. A woman consults you at her booking visit in her second pregnancy at 12 weeks as she wishes to discuss delivery. She sustained a third-degree tear after a lift-out forceps in her first pregnancy. How would you advise her?
    *See Chapter 36, Perineal trauma.*

39. A premature infant is delivered at 28 weeks' gestation. Outline the important principles involved in maximizing outcome in the first few minutes.
    *See Chapter 38, Neonatal resuscitation.*

40. How does knowledge of the physiological adaptations the newborn infant undergoes influence your approach to resuscitation in neonates?
    *See Chapter 38, Neonatal resuscitation.*

41. The routine newborn examination is an important screening tool in the first few days of life. Discuss.
    *See Chapter 39, Common neonatal problems.*

42. A 26-year-old woman has just delivered a 5.0 kg baby. As the obstetric registrar on call, you are urgently summoned to the labour suite. When you arrive in the room, the woman is shocked, the blood loss is 100 mL, and your differential diagnosis includes an inverted uterus. Detail the management of this woman.

    *See Chapter 41, Postpartum collapse.*

43. Describe the management of a patient with retained placenta.

    *See Chapter 42, Postpartum haemorrhage.*

44. A 19-year-old woman who is 8 days postnatal, having undergone an emergency caesarean section for failure to progress, is admitted with a pyrexia of 38.5°C. Discuss the possible diagnoses and her subsequent management.

    *See Chapter 43, Postpartum pyrexia.*

45. Discuss the possible psychiatric sequelae of pregnancy and how these might be prevented or treated.

    *See Chapter 44, Disturbed mood.*

46. With references to specific examples, outline the benefits and risks of breastfeeding to the mother and the newborn infant. Utilizing the same examples, also demonstrate how rates of breastfeeding can be maximized.

    *See Chapter 45, Problems with breastfeeding.*

# GYNAECOLOGY

47. You have delivered a baby with ambiguous genitalia. How is this problem managed?
    *See Chapter 46, Normal and abnormal development of the genitalia.*

48. An 18-year-old presents with primary amenorrhoea. How will you try to establish the cause of this from the history and examination? Discuss which investigations would be appropriate.
    *See Chapter 48, Menarche and adolescent gynaecology.*

49. Briefly discuss the recent advances and possible future developments in contraception.
    *See Chapter 50, Contraception, sterilization and termination of pregnancy.*

50. A 49-year-old woman presents at the gynaecology clinic. On examination, she is found to have a 16-week-sized fibroid uterus. Discuss the management of this patient.
    *See Chapter 51.2, Uterine fibroids and menorrhagia.*

51. How should menorrhagia be investigated and treated?
    *See Chapter 51.3, Heavy and irregular menstruation.*

52. A 16-year-old girl presents to the gynaecology clinic as she is suffering from painful periods that are not relieved by aspirin. Discuss the logical steps in the diagnostic process and the treatment options available.
    *See Chapter 51.4, Dysmenorrhoea.*

53. What is the clinical presentation of endometriosis? How would you manage infertility associated with endometriosis?
    *See Chapter 51.5, Endometriosis and gonadotrophin releasing hormone analogues.*

54. Discuss the diagnosis and management options of premenstrual tension?
    *See Chapter 51.7, Premenstrual syndrome.*

55. Discuss the management of tubal disease as a cause of infertility.
    *See Chapter 52.2, Female infertility.*

56. Semen analysis is a laboratory investigation with an inherently low sensitivity and specificity. Discuss.
    *See Chapter 52.3, Male infertility.*

57. The latest advances in assisted reproduction technology have led to a significant increase in multiple pregnancy rates, especially high-order ones. This is an iatrogenic problem that should be dealt with effectively. Discuss.
    *See Chapter 52.4, Assisted reproduction.*

58. Discuss the clinical manifestations, diagnosis and management of polycystic ovarian syndrome.
    *See Chapter 53, Polycystic ovarian syndrome.*

59. Critically appraise the treatment options available for hirsutism.
    *See Chapter 54, Hirsutism and virilism.*

60. Discuss the various steps in the investigation of an 18-year-old student who has failed to commence menstruation. She has otherwise normal secondary sexual characteristics and no obvious abnormalities on general examination.
    *See Chapter 55, Amenorrhoea and oligomenorrhoea.*

61. A 55-year-old woman with severe hot flushes and night sweats presents in the gynaecology clinic. She had a lumpectomy and radiotherapy for breast cancer 4 years previously. Her mother is wheelchair-bound because of severe osteoporosis. Discuss the treatment options and justify your management.
    *See Chapter 56, Menopause and hormone replacement therapy.*

62. A 25-year-old nulliparous woman presents with 7 weeks of amenorrhoea and a positive home pregnancy test. She has experienced abdominal pain and vaginal spotting of blood for 24 hours. Discuss the differential diagnosis and investigation and briefly outline the treatments available.
    *See Chapter 57, Problems in early pregnancy.*

63. A 32-year-old woman complaining of recurrent episodes of cystitis, which occur once or twice a month, is referred by her general practitioner. Describe your initial assessment and subsequent management.
    *See Chapter 61, Lower urinary tract infections.*

64. A 67-year-old woman presents with a history of symptomatic prolapse and occasional stress incontinence whilst coughing and sneezing. On examination by her general practitioner, she was found to have second-degree uterine descent, a moderate cystocele and mild rectocele. Describe your subsequent management.
    *See Chapter 62, Urogenital prolapse.*

65. Describe the management of a 15-year-old girl attending the casualty department with lower abdominal pain and offensive vaginal discharge who is systemically unwell.
    *See Chapter 63.1, Infection and sexual health.*

66. A 22-year-old woman attends your outpatient clinic, referred with an offensive vaginal discharge. She has confided to the nurse that she also has some 'lumps' on the vulva. Outline your management.
   *See Chapter 63.1, Infection and sexual health.*

67. A married couple presents to the gynaecology clinic with 4 years of infertility. All preliminary investigations in primary care have been normal. During the consultation, the woman bursts into tears and admits that consummation of the marriage has never taken place. Describe what you will do next.
   *See Chapter 63.2, Dyspareunia and other psychosexual problems.*

68. A 14-year-old girl is referred to your clinic with heavy periods. During the consultation she appears very withdrawn and tearful. She asks to be put on 'the pill' and urges you not to tell her mother, who has temporarily left the room. What sort of issues does this presentation raise and how would you manage them?
   *See Chapter 63.3, Child sex abuse.*

69. You are the on-call specialist registrar in obstetrics and gynaecology and a 32-year-old woman is referred to you by the police with a history of alleged rape and vaginal bleeding. There is no forensic medical officer available to examine this woman and you are asked to perform a forensic medical examination of the complainant and to treat her injuries. Discuss how would you manage this problem.
   *See Chapter 63.4, Rape and rape counselling.*

70. A 54-year-old woman has a 3-year history of persistent pruritus vulvae that has failed to respond to repeated antifungal treatment and hydrocortisone creams. She has no history of atopy or vaginal discharge. General examination was unremarkable. On pelvic examination, the vulval skin had a parchment-like appearance, with some areas of telangiectases and loss of the normal architecture. What is the differential diagnosis? Explain which one is most likely and discuss how you would manage this problem.
   *See Chapter 64, Benign vulval problems.*

71. Counsel a woman who has been given a diagnosis of vulval vestibulitis.
   *See Chapter 65, Vulval pain syndromes.*

72. A 26-year-old nulliparous woman has had her second-ever cervical smear and this has been reported as moderate dyskaryosis. She is currently using combined oral contraception and is normal on examination apart from a cervical ectropion. Describe an appropriate management plan and what would be appropriate counselling for this woman.
   *See Chapter 66, Pre-invasive disease.*

73. A 54-year-old woman presents with postmenopausal bleeding. She has been on tamoxifen for 2 years following treatment for a node-positive breast cancer. This tumour was oestrogen-receptor positive. Discuss her further management.
   *See Chapter 67, Endometrial cancer.*

74. Describe the management of a 26-year-old nulliparous woman referred by a practice nurse with a cervical smear report suggesting high-grade dyskaryosis suspicious of invasive disease.

    *See Chapter 68, Cervical cancer.*

75. A 25-year-old nulliparous woman presents with a tender mass arising from the pelvis and consistent in size with a 16-week gestation. Pregnancy test is negative. Ultrasound scan confirms the presence of a complex ovarian mass with features highly suspicious of malignancy. The eventual histology is that of a germ-cell tumour. Describe your management.

    *See Chapter 69, Benign and malignant ovarian masses.*

76. Describe the management of a 67-year-old woman presenting with a 4-week history of a painful 3.5 cm vulval ulcer close to the clitoris.

    *See Chapter 70, Vulval and vaginal cancer.*

77. Describe the acute gynaecological management of suspected molar pregnancy.

    *See Chapter 71, Gestational trophoblastic disease.*

# OBSTETRICS

1. **A 32-year-old multiparous women presents at 10 weeks' gestation to the antenatal clinic. She has a blood pressure of 140/90 mmHg. Outline the management of this problem.**

- If repeat blood pressure measurements give similar values, these levels of blood pressure indicate pre-existing or chronic hypertension. Although the majority of these cases will represent essential hypertension, the remaining cases will be secondary to other causes.

  **(2 marks)**

- A careful history should be elicited, including any family history of hypertension, a history suggestive of possible secondary causes, and whether any anti-hypertensive agents are already being taken.

  **(2 marks)**

- Agents with known detrimental effects on the fetus – such as either angiotensin-converting enzyme (ACE) inhibitors or diuretics – should be stopped and an alternative anti-hypertensive agent considered.

  **(2 marks)**

- On examination, fundoscopy should be undertaken to assess the severity of the hypertension. With mild hypertension, A-V nipping would be expected; however, exudates and haemorrhages suggest a more severe picture.

  **(2 marks)**

- Investigations should include a full blood count, urea and electrolytes, liver function tests (LFTs) and a 24-hour urinary protein determination.

  **(2 marks)**

- *Essential hypertension* normally presents with little in the history; however, there may well be a family history and the woman may already be having anti-hypertensive treatment.

  **(2 marks)**

- The most common *secondary causes* of hypertension are those of the renal diseases. These include autosomal dominant polycystic kidney disease. Chronic pyelonephritis may present with nocturia, recurrent urinary tract infections (UTIs) and childhood enuresis. Investigations should include an ultrasound scan of the kidneys and a determination of urea and electrolytes. Adrenal causes are rare but need to be considered. Conn's disease will present with hypertension, hypokalaemia and hypernatraemia. Treatment is with anti-hypertensive agents and potassium supplementation. A phaeochromocytoma is another rare cause of secondary hypertension and may present with transient bouts of hypertension and palpitations; 24-hour urinary determination of catecholamines and vanillylmandelic acid (VMA) will confirm the diagnosis.                                                   **(3 marks)**

- Treatment should be aimed at controlling the blood pressure. In mild hypertensive disease, treatment has not been shown to be beneficial to fetal outcome. Drugs that have been used include *methyldopa*, which is safe in terms of the fetus but may cause abnormal LFTs and depression, *labetolol*, which has been shown to cause fetal and neonatal bradycardias, and *nifedipine*. These drugs can be used as single agents or in combination.                                                   **(2 marks)**

- Careful antenatal surveillance is essential, as there is a 20 per cent risk of superimposed pre-eclampsia; this should include regular blood pressure and urinary dipstick testing. Platelet count and uric acid estimations may be an adjunct to this screening, as they have been shown to change prior to the onset of proteinuria. Ultrasound assessment of the fetal growth should be undertaken at intervals throughout pregnancy.    **(3 marks)**

*See Chapter 6.1, Chronic hypertension.*

## 2. Evaluate the methods of fetal assessment in a woman with insulin-dependent diabetes mellitus diagnosed 3 years before conception.

- Early ultrasound assessment of the fetus should occur at or around 6 weeks' gestation; this allows both accurate dating and confirmation of an ongoing pregnancy. **(2 marks)**

- Serum screening for Down's syndrome is problematic in pregnancies complicated by maternal diabetes as the serum alpha-fetoprotein (aFP) levels are reduced. It is probably preferable to offer ultrasound nuchal translucency (NT) screening, as this is unaffected by diabetes. **(4 marks)**

- A mid-trimester anomaly scan should be arranged to exclude identifiable cardiac, renal or neural tube defects; these abnormalities are more common in women with diabetes. **(2 marks)**

- Although sacral agenesis is a relatively uncommon abnormality, it does have a very strong association with diabetes. However, it should be noted that the detection rate is in the order of 50 per cent and so a normal scan does not exclude a structural abnormality. **(2 marks)**

- Serial scans should be arranged from 26 weeks' gestation to exclude both fetal macrosomia and polyhydramnios. Both of these pregnancy complications are indications of poor maternal glucose control and may affect the perinatal outcome – increasing the rates of shoulder dystocia and preterm delivery respectively. The serial scans are also indicated on the basis of an increased risk of fetal growth restriction. **(4 marks)**

- There is an increased incidence of unexplained stillbirths after 36 weeks' gestation in pregnancies complicated by maternal diabetes; this merits extra vigilance. **(2 marks)**

- Many schemes have been suggested, and these include kick charts, non-stress cardiotograms (CTGs), liquor volume, and umbilical artery Doppler waveform analyses. However, when subjected to randomized controlled trials (RCTs), none of these investigations has been shown to influence perinatal mortality. **(4 marks)**

*See Chapter 6.2, Diabetes mellitus.*

**3. A 24-year-old woman with poorly controlled insulin-dependent diabetes attends a pre-pregnancy clinic. Justify the advice specific to her condition that you would give.**

- She should be advised that poor glucose control in pregnancy increases the risk of congenital anomalies five-fold, and also increases the risk of miscarriage. However, with good control (as suggested by an HbA1c estimation <6.5 per cent), these risks approximate to those of women without diabetes.                          **(4 marks)**

- The importance of good control should be stressed without alarming the woman. Even with poor control, most women with diabetes will not have a congenitally abnormal baby.                                                                                  **(2 marks)**

- It should be explained that an ultrasound scan at approximately 20 weeks' gestation will examine for structural anomalies – particularly those affecting the fetal heart, kidneys and central nervous system.                                                          **(2 marks)**

- She should be informed that although the chromosomal abnormality rate remains constant, serum screening tests are affected by diabetes, and ultrasound NT screening is preferable.                                                                               **(2 marks)**

- She should be advised to continue on a suitable diet and be referred to a diabetic nurse and dietician. Rubella status should be checked, and folic acid prescribed. Contraceptive measures should be offered until good control is attained.                          **(2 marks)**

- Glucose should be kept below 5.5 mmol/L (fasting) and less than 7 mmol/L (post-meals). Insulin requirements go up during pregnancy and require careful monitoring. She should monitor her own blood sugar levels pre-meal and post-meal, and have blood taken for HbA1c to monitor long-term control. She is at increased risk of both diabetic keto-acidosis and hypoglycaemia and should be educated about the signs and symptoms of both complications.                                                                      **(3 marks)**

- There is also a risk that both diabetic nephropathy and retinopathy will worsen with pregnancy, and baseline renal function tests should be performed. However, these complications usually improve post-delivery. There is an increased risk of pre-eclampsia, which will require regular monitoring of blood pressure and urine.                      **(2 marks)**

- There is an increased risk of polyhydramnios and this is associated with an increase in premature delivery. Poor control is associated with macrosomia and an increased rate of shoulder dystocia. The unexplained stillbirth rate is increased after 36 weeks, thus careful fetal monitoring will be necessary.                                             **(3 marks)**

*See Chapter 6.2, Diabetes mellitus.*

**4. A 26-year-old Asian woman attends an antenatal booking clinic. In the referral letter it is highlighted that she has an atrial septal heart lesion. Outline the subsequent management.**

- This is the most common congenital heart lesion in the UK. It is normally well tolerated in pregnancy and the maternal mortality from this lesion is less than 1 per cent. Therefore the patient can be reassured of a good pregnancy outcome.   **(2 marks)**

- Antenatal care needs to focus initially on the maternal considerations. It should be ascertained from the history whether this is her first pregnancy and, if not, whether complications from the lesion worsened in previous pregnancies.   **(2 marks)**

- It should also be ascertained whether the lesion has been surgically corrected, as those that have been corrected are associated with a better prognosis. The history should enable determination of whether there are any functional prognostic indicators, such as those of the New York Heart Association, or the presence of pulmonary hypertension.   **(2 marks)**

- It should be appreciated that there is an increased risk of the fetus having a congenital heart abnormality, and that this ranges from 3 to 10 per cent. Prenatal diagnosis of more serious conditions is possible with high-resolution ultrasound at 22 weeks. This should be offered to the couple as a screening mechanism, but it should be made clear that it does not identify all cardiac lesions.   **(3 marks)**

- Antenatal care should take place in a multidisciplinary setting with a cardiologist available. If the lesion has not been surgically corrected, an echocardiogram is of use to determine the extent of the defect. At each antenatal visit, assessments should be made to exclude supraventricular tachycardias, right heart failure and pulmonary hypertension. If these do present, they should be treated in consultation with the cardiologist. If there is any evidence of maternal chronic hypoxia (pulmonary hypertension), fetal growth assessment is mandatory.   **(5 marks)**

- There is no indication for routine induction of labour unless there are obstetric indications. A caesarean section should only be performed for obstetric indications.   **(1 mark)**

- The woman should receive prophylactic antibiotics.   **(1 mark)**

- Labour should be conducted in the left lateral position and adequate analgesia given to avoid stress.   **(1 mark)**

- A continuous electrocardiogram (ECG) should be used to monitor for arrhythmias, and any arrhythmias should be treated.   **(1 mark)**

- Ergometrine should be avoided as it can cause dramatic changes in haemodynamic status. **(1 mark)**

- Fluid overload should be avoided. **(1 mark)**

  *See Chapter 6.3, Cardiac disease.*

**5. Discuss the management of a 34-year-old woman with a known history of Graves' disease who is contemplating pregnancy.**

- A full medical history should be taken to determine whether this woman has been treated for her hyperthyroidism and whether the disease is well controlled. **(2 marks)**

- Medical 'block and replace' treatments may have been initiated; these involve complete suppression of thyroid function with propylthiouracil (PTU) or carbimazole and then replacement with thyroxine. The use of 'block and replace' treatment regimens has no place in the therapy of pregnant women due to the risk of fetal hypothyroidism. Therefore, all women contemplating pregnancy should be switched to a 'blocking-only' regimen, involving suppression with PTU or carbimazole. The woman should be offered contraceptive measures until she is euthyroid. **(3 marks)**

- Radioactive iodine may have been used as a curative or diagnostic procedure, and if this is the case, pregnancy should be deferred for at least 1 year after treatment, because of the increased risk of a congenital abnormality. **(2 marks)**

- The woman may have undergone a total or partial surgical thyroidectomy, which has rendered her either euthyroid or hypothyroid and on replacement therapy. **(2 marks)**

- Although the mother may have been treated for her Graves' disease, she will have circulating antibodies to thyroid tissue. The level of these antibodies should be determined. In the treated mother, a low antibody titre is associated with a low risk of fetal hyperthyroidism. However, these antibodies can cross the placenta and cause fetal hyperthyroidism after 20 weeks' gestation (when the fetal thyroid becomes active). **(3 marks)**

- Fetal hyperthyroidism is associated with premature labour, hydrops fetalis, polyhydramnios and a fetal goitre. The presentation of fetal hyperthyroidism can involve any of these complications or a fetal tachycardia of >180 bpm. **(2 marks)**

- Treatment options for fetal hyperthyroidism are dependent on gestation. If the fetus is near term, delivery is an option. However, if it is remote from term, maternal PTU therapy can be commenced; PTU crosses the placenta. Maternal thyroxine, which does not cross the placenta, can be given to counteract the effects of PTU on the mother. **(2 marks)**

- Throughout the pregnancy, thyroid function tests should be repeated at 3-monthly intervals and, if the woman is taking thyroxine replacement therapy, the aim should be to keep the free thyroxine level in the normal range. If thyroid function tests have been stable prior to pregnancy, adjustment will rarely be required. **(4 marks)**

*See Chapter 6.4, Thyroid disease.*

**6. A 25-year-old nulliparous woman has a repeat full blood count at 28 weeks' gestation confirming a platelet count of 65 $\times 10^9$/L. Outline your differential diagnosis and antenatal management.**

- The initial differential diagnosis includes:
  gestational thrombocytopenia
  idiopathic thrombocytopenic purpura
  other immune conditions – systemic lupus erythematosus (SLE), antiphospholipid
    syndrome
  pre-eclampsia
  viral infection
  haematological malignancy.                                       **(6 marks)**

- The first step is to take the relevant history. It is important to establish whether she has noted epistaxis, menorrhagia, or bleeding after dental or surgical procedures – either prior to or during the pregnancy. A history of any medication that might predispose to a thrombocytopenia (e.g. heparin or trimethoprim) should be noted. Any family history of a bleeding tendency should be sought. A recent history of flu-like symptoms, illness or headache would suggest a viral infection.                         **(3 marks)**

- In addition to measurement of blood pressure and urinary dipstick testing, a detailed examination should be performed – particularly for:
  petechiae – most typically on dependent regions of body (lower limbs/feet), over the
    site of trauma (top of shoes, under a blood pressure cuff) and in the mouth
  any bruising
  any bleeding gums, especially prevalent after brushing teeth.      **(2 marks)**

- Investigations should include a full blood count (it is important to compare this to the count performed at the booking visit), a peripheral blood film, assessment of clotting status, renal and liver function tests and urate level, determination of the presence/absence of lupus anticoagulant/anticardiolipin antibodies (aCL) and antiplatelet antibodies, and a virology screen – Epstein–Barr virus (EBV), cytomegalovirus (CMV), human immunodeficiency virus (HIV).        **(3 marks)**

- Fetal growth, well-being and liquor volume should be assessed by an ultrasound scan.
                                                                    **(1 mark)**

- The woman should be reviewed 1 week later, in order to review results and repeat the blood count – to ensure that the platelet count is not decreasing rapidly. (Bone marrow aspiration may need to be considered in severe thrombocytopenia or if there is a rapid fall in the platelet count.) It is sensible to obtain help and advice from a haematologist, and review by an anaesthetist is required in the antenatal period. The neonatologists should be informed of the possibility of complications affecting the baby.    **(2 marks)**

- In general, unless the platelet count falls below $50 \times 10^9$/L, or she develops symptoms, management should be expectant. **(1 mark)**

- If the platelet count falls below $50 \times 10^9$/L, corticosteroid therapy should be considered. An IgG infusion may be required if there is a poor response to corticosteroids. **(1 mark)**

- Nearer term, a management plan for delivery needs to be documented. In general, a vaginal delivery is not contraindicated, and regional anaesthesia is permitted if the platelet count is $80 \times 10^9$/L. **(1 mark)**

  *See Chapter 6.5, Haematological conditions.*

**7. Pulmonary embolism remains a major cause of maternal death. Outline the steps that should be taken to minimize the risk of thromboembolism in pregnant women.**

- The risks of thromboembolism are increased from early in the first trimester until the late puerperium. **(2 marks)**

- Close attention should be given to any women presenting with leg or chest symptoms compatible with thrombosis. These symptoms require prompt investigation. **(2 marks)**

- Women with a history of thrombotic episodes or known thrombophilia should be considered for heparin prophylaxis throughout pregnancy and the puerperium. **(2 marks)**

- Women with multiple risk factors during pregnancy should be considered for thromboprophylaxis during pregnancy. **(2 marks)**

- All women undergoing caesarean section should be assessed for risk.
  Low risk-women – i.e. with no risk factors – require early mobilization and adequate hydration.
  Moderate-risk women – defined as having one to two risk factors: age >35 years, weight >80 kg, para 4 or more, gross varicose veins, current infection, pre-eclampsia, etc. – should be managed as above, but with the addition of thromboembolic deterrent (TED) stockings and heparin prophylaxis.
  High-risk women – defined as having three or more moderate factors, a personal family history of venous thromboembolism (VTE), major intercurrent disease, known thrombophilia or undergoing a caesarean hysterectomy – require heparin prophylaxis. **(6 marks)**

- Aspirin has no fetal side effects; however, there is the potential for maternal gastrointestinal bleeding. Low-molecular-weight heparin has no fetal side effects as it does not cross the placenta, and there is no evidence of maternal osteoporosis with long-term maternal use.
  Warfarin is teratotogenic to the fetus throughout pregnancy and therefore should not be used antenatally. **(4 marks)**

- Women with a history of VTE should receive anticoagulant prophylaxis from at least 6 weeks following delivery. Heparin or warfarin may be used. Low-molecular-weight heparin has the advantage of once-daily administration and it has no effect on bone mineral density. **(2 marks)**

*See Chapter 6.5, Haematological conditions, and Chapter 9, Maternal mortality.*

**8. A 34-year-old woman with polycystic kidneys seeks your advice as she wishes to become pregnant. Routine blood tests demonstrate that she has serum creatinine of 175 μmol/L. How would you advise her with regard to pregnancy?**

- The women should be advised about healthy living, and folic acid should be prescribed. Her rubella status should be checked and immunization should be given if she is not immune.                                                        **(2 marks)**

- She should be advised that there is increased risk of miscarriage, pre-eclampsia, intrauterine growth restriction (IUGR), premature delivery, caesarean section and perinatal mortality.                                                    **(4 marks)**

- She should be aware that the main factors that affect fetal outcome are the severities of renal impairment, hypertension and proteinuria.                          **(2 marks)**

- She should also be advised of an increased risk of further loss of maternal renal function. In a woman with a serum creatinine of 175 μmol/L, this risk is between 25 and 50 per cent.                                                                       **(2 marks)**

- She should be advised that polycystic kidney is an autosomal dominant condition and that there is a 50 per cent chance of transmission to offspring.           **(2 marks)**

- Sixty per cent of the infants of women with moderate renal impairment (such as in this case) are born prematurely.                                              **(2 marks)**

- Careful monitoring of blood pressure is essential, as good control prevents deterioration in renal impairment and improves fetal outcome. Blood pressure control can be achieved with labetolol, nifedipine and methyldopa. Many patients with chronic renal disease need combination anti-hypertensive therapies.                            **(2 marks)**

- Serial growth scans and umbilical artery Doppler are indicated from 24 weeks in view of the high risk of IUGR. There is also an increased risk of polyhydramnios if the blood urea is >10 mmol/L, and fetal death is increased if the blood urea is >25 mmol/L.   **(2 marks)**

- Maternal admission to hospital should be considered if hypertension becomes marked or there is evidence of superimposed pre-eclampsia.                          **(2 marks)**

*See Chapter 6.6, Renal disease.*

## 9. A 37-year-old woman who is known to have systemic lupus erythematosus presents at the antenatal clinic. Outline the management of this pregnancy.

- A full obstetric history should be taken. It should be ascertained whether she is in remission or has ongoing active disease, which is requiring treatment. **(2 marks)**

- A treatment history should be sought to determine the drugs that the patient is taking. Hydroxychloroquine can be continued, as it is safe in pregnancy and withdrawal may precipitate flare. It also has a very long half-life, such that the fetus remains exposed for up to 3 months after the mother discontinues the drug. Prednisolone and azathioprine are also safe to continue in pregnancy. **(2 marks)**

- Basic investigations should include a full blood count to ascertain whether she has anaemia associated with chronic disease, which will require treatment, or a haemolytic anaemia. Urea and electrolytes should be measured to determine her renal function, as these have a close correlation with the obstetric outcome. Blood should also be taken for autoantibodies, the commonest being antinuclear antibody (96 per cent). Anti-Ro and anti-La antibodies should also be measured, as these determine the risk of the fetus developing postnatal problems. **(4 marks)**

- The woman should be counselled that if SLE is quiescent, there is no renal involvement, and if she is Ro/La and antiphospholipid (aPL) negative, there is no adverse effect of the disease on the pregnancy. Active disease at conception, renal involvement and antiphospholipid syndrome (APS) increase the risks of miscarriage, pre-eclampsia, IUGR, premature delivery and stillbirth. **(2 marks)**

- In a 37-year-old woman, screening for Down's syndrome should also be discussed. **(1 mark)**

- The management of this pregnancy should occur within a multidisciplinary setting. There is a 40–60 per cent chance of a flare during pregnancy and this should be treated with either the introduction of corticosteriods or an increase in the dose. Azathiaprine may need to be introduced in cases of resistance. **(2 marks)**

- Hypertension should be treated with labetolol, nifedipine or methyldopa. Serial urea and electrolyte measurements should be made in cases in which there is evidence of renal compromise. Deterioration in renal function may necessitate delivery of the fetus. **(2 marks)**

- In patients who are having any form of treatment of hypertension or flares, serial growth scans should be commenced from 24 weeks, as there is an increased incidence of IUGR within this group. **(2 marks)**

- In patients who are anti-Ro antibody positive, there is a risk of the fetus developing congenital heart block or neonatal cutaneous discoid lupus. Congenital heart block occurs in 2 per cent of women with anti-Ro antibodies, most commonly between 18 and 30 weeks' gestation, and is permanent and normally requires postnatal cardiac pacing. Discoid lupus develops within the first 2 weeks of life as geographical lesions and usually resolves within 6 months. **(3 marks)**

*See Chapter 6.7, Autoimmune conditions.*

**10. A 24-year-old primiparous woman presents to the accident and emergency department with persistent vomiting when 7 weeks pregnant. Outline the management of this woman.**

- Vomiting is a common feature of pregnancy (approximately 50 per cent). Most cases will settle before 14–16 weeks without treatment. Only a small percentage (1 per cent) of women will have classical hyperemesis gravidarum, which is defined as vomiting within pregnancy that causes alterations in urea and electrolytes and liver function parameters.                                                                    **(3 marks)**

- A full history should be taken to determine the severity of the vomiting and to exclude other causes of vomiting in early pregnancy; these include UTIs, diabetes, hepatitis and, rarely, Addison's disease.                                                             **(2 marks)**

- A clinical examination should assess how dehydrated she is. Investigations should include the measurement of urea and electrolytes (which may demonstrate hyponatraemia, hypokalaemia and a high serum urea), liver function tests (which may reveal mildly elevated transaminases and bilirubin levels), and a random blood glucose (to exclude diabetes). Thyroid function tests will be abnormal in approximately 70 per cent of cases. A full blood count will demonstrate an increased haematocrit (in keeping with the picture of dehydration). Urinary dipstick testing may indicate a UTI and/or the presence of ketones. An ultrasound scan should be arranged to confirm a singleton pregnancy and to exclude a hydatidiform mole or a multiple pregnancy, both of which are associated with increased vomiting in pregnancy.                            **(6 marks)**

- If it is not adequately treated, hyperemesis gravidarum carries risks to the mother. These include Wernicke's encephalopathy, peripheral neuropathy, hyponatraemia, Mallory–Weis tears, malnutrition and thrombosis.                                           **(3 marks)**

- The most common fetal complication of hyperemesis is IUGR. A 40 per cent fetal loss rate is associated with Wernicke's encephalopathy.                              **(2 marks)**

- Treatment should include admission to hospital. Intravenous fluid replacement should be started; however, dextrose should be avoided, as it increases the likelihood of Wernicke's encephalopathy and other central nervous system problems. Thiamine supplementation should be initiated if vomiting continues despite treatment. If simple hydration is ineffective, anti-emetics such as cyclizine (50 mg b.d.) or domperidone (10 mg b.d.) can be used. If these agents fail to resolve the vomiting, corticosteroids (prednisolone 40–50 mg o.d.) have been shown to be effective. Prophylactic heparin should be considered if vomiting persists.                                                              **(4 marks)**

*See Chapter 6.8, Liver and gastrointestinal disease.*

**11. A 26-year-old woman who is 36 weeks pregnant in her first pregnancy presents to the antenatal clinic with a skin rash. Briefly outline the possible differential diagnoses and how these conditions could be treated.**

- The differential diagnosis should include:
  - pre-existing dermatological diseases – contact dermatitis, eczema, psoriasis
  - pregnancy-specific disorders – polymorphic eruption of pregnancy (PEP), pemphigoid gestationis, prurigo of pregnancy
  - systemic disorders – systemic lupus infections and Stevens–Johnson syndrome.

**(6 marks)**

- A full dermatological history will differentiate between contact dermatitis, eczema and psoriasis.

  Contact dermatitis may have been coincident to a change in washing powder, soap etc. Treatment is reassurance and removal of the stimulant; mild topical steroids (1 per cent hydrocortisone) may be given for symptomatic relieve.

  Eczema will have been present prior to the onset of pregnancy. The rash is usually localized to the flexural aspects. There may also have been a history of atopy as a child. Treatment with bland emollients and topical steroids is safe in pregnancy.

  Psoriasis may present for the first time during pregnancy. The rash is also initially in the flexural areas. Treatments including coal tar and dithranol are safe in pregnancy, but methotrexate is contraindicated. **(3 marks)**

- The most common pregnancy-specific disorder is PEP. It usually presents in the third trimester of pregnancy with a pruritic urticarial rash that has umbilical sparing. It has no effect on the fetal outcome, and treatment is symptomatic, with the application of 1 per cent methonal in aqueous cream and antihistamines. Occasionally topical steroids may be required. **(2 marks)**

- Prurigo of pregnancy is the next most common pregnancy-specific disorder. However, it is more common in multiparous patients. It resolves after pregnancy and treatment is the same as for PEP. **(2 marks)**

- Phemphigoid gestationalis is the rarest of the dermatoses of pregnancy. It can present at any time within pregnancy with pruritic, urticated erythematous papules without umbilical sparing. It has been associated with low-birth-weight infants and prematurity. **(2 marks)**

- The most common systemic conditions that may affect the pregnant women are infections. Chicken pox is one cause of a global body rash, presenting with an urticarial pustular rash. If diagnosed after 20 weeks and within 24 hours of the rash presenting, oral aciclovir should be given. Rubella and parvovirus are other causes of a rash that may present in pregnancy. Parvovirus presents with a classical red rash on the cheeks; infection late in pregnancy has little effect on the fetus. Rubella presents with a global maculopapular rash; at this stage in pregnancy it has not been shown to have any adverse effects on the fetus. **(3 marks)**

- A rare but important rash that needs to be excluded is that of Stevens–Johnson syndrome. It is normally related to an adverse drug reaction or infection, and cessation of the stimulus is required. Systemic lupus erythematosus is also a rare cause of a facial rash that may present in pregnancy. **(2 marks)**

  *See Chapter 6.11, Dermatological conditions.*

**12. A 22-year-old ex-intravenous drug abuser (currently on methadone) books at 15 weeks in her first pregnancy. She is hepatitis B positive. Outline a comprehensive plan for her care.**

- At the booking visit, it is important to establish all the legal and illicit drugs that the woman is using; confirmation can be obtained by sending urine for toxicology assessment. The amount of methadone currently used should be documented, with the name of the chemist supplying the methadone (if she is admitted to hospital, the chemist needs to be informed to stop the prescription). **(2 marks)**

- The advantages and disadvantages of reducing methadone in pregnancy need to be discussed. The advantages include decreased withdrawal symptoms in neonates if methadone is discontinued before 36 weeks. The disadvantage is that the reduced dose can lead to the temptation to 'top-up' the methadone with illicit drug use. The need to avoid supplementing methadone with illicit drugs should be stressed. **(2 marks)**

- Routine booking bloods should include testing for hepatitis C and HIV. A full screen for sexually transmitted diseases (STDs) should be performed. In view of her hepatitis-B-positive status, infectivity should be determined by analysis of her serology. Full testing of her partner should be encouraged, with referral to the drug liaison service if appropriate. **(2 marks)**

- Throughout the pregnancy, there should be full multidisciplinary involvement. This will include the named consultant, a specialist midwife, drug liaison services, the community midwife, the general practitioner and, depending on co-existent disease, an infectious disease physician. The potential need for social service involvement should also be assessed. A consultant paediatrician should be alerted to potential neonatal complications. If venous access problems are anticipated (antenatally or in labour), the assistance of a consultant anaesthetist should be sought. Similarly, a management plan relating to analgesia in labour should be developed in advance. **(3 marks)**

- There should be a low threshold for ultrasound estimations of fetal growth because drug users are at a higher risk of IUGR due to associated social deprivation, poor nutrition and often associated high nicotine intake. In addition, attendance for an ultrasound scan provides opportunities to see these women more frequently (they are often poor clinic attenders). **(2 marks)**

- During the labour, methadone should be prescribed and not omitted. All methods of pain relief can be offered in labour, although cyclizine should be avoided as this may potentiate the effects of illicit drugs. It is important to recognize that these women often require greater amounts of pain relief than normal. **(2 marks)**

- As she is hepatitis B positive, there should be the shortest duration possible between membranes rupturing and delivery, early recourse to Syntocinon, avoidance of fetal blood sampling, and delivery by the least traumatic method.                    **(2 marks)**

- After delivery, the baby should be observed for signs of drug withdrawal; admission to the special care baby unit is not routine. The mother should stay in for 5–10 days postpartum to remain with the baby whilst it is being observed.                    **(2 marks)**

- As the mother is hepatitis B positive, appropriate administration of hepatitis B immunoglobulin/vaccine should be prescribed.                    **(1 mark)**

- Throughout the antenatal, intrapartum and postnatal care, confidentiality is of paramount importance. It is particularly important to be careful about what is documented in the hand-held notes.                    **(2 marks)**

*See Chapter 6.12, Drug and alcohol misuse, and Chapter 7.4, Infection.*

## 13. Justify the statement 'all women who smoke and are pregnant should be offered a programme for cessation of smoking'.

- Smoking in pregnancy is a common problem; the reported incidence in the UK is 27 per cent of pregnant women. Although it is often difficult to distinguish the effects of smoking from those of confounding variables, smoking has short-term and long-term effects on both the fetus and the mother.                                              **(2 marks)**

- *Maternal.* Smoking in pregnancy increases the risk of postoperative chest infections and venous thromboemboli (particularly following operative deliveries). Female smoking increases the risk of lung cancer and cardiovascular disease later in life. There is evidence that both ovarian function and implantation may be affected by smoking, thus reducing the fertility of these women – the risk of miscarriage is also increased.                          **(4 marks)**

- *Fetal.* Short-term fetal effects include a doubling of the risk of premature delivery, and a consequent increase in perinatal mortality. This increased premature delivery rate is, at least in part, related to iatrogenic delivery for placental abruption and praevia, both of which are associated with smoking. Smoking in pregnancy is associated with lower birth weight for gestation.                                                       **(4 marks)**

- The long-term effects of in-utero exposure to maternal smoking are confounded by childhood effects of parental smoking. However, it appears that cognitive performance is reduced in children whose mothers smoked in pregnancy.                          **(2 marks)**

- Although the majority of the effects of smoking in pregnancy are detrimental, interestingly smoking appears to have a protective effect on the incidence of pre-eclampsia. Any positive effects are greatly outweighed by the negative effects.                          **(3 marks)**

- Standard advice from obstetricians and midwives has little effect on the outcome measures of premature delivery and birth weight. However, smoking cessation programmes do show significant improvements in both the preterm delivery rate and birth weight. Self-help material has some benefit in approximately 4 per cent of smokers. The effectiveness and safety of nicotine replacement therapy in pregnancy have yet to be established.                                                       **(5 marks)**

*See Chapter 6.13, Smoking.*

**14. A 25-year-old woman in her fourth pregnancy is seen in the booking clinic at 20 weeks' gestation. Her community midwife has taken routine bloods. Her haemoglobin concentration is 7.2 g/dL. How would you manage her pregnancy?**

- A full history should be obtained. This should include ethnic origin, as certain forms of anaemia are more common in particular ethnic minorities. A dietary history should be elicited to determine whether the patient has a poor iron intake. The pregnancy interval should be noted, as a short pregnancy interval predisposes to iron deficiency anaemia.

    **(2 marks)**

- A full blood count should be taken. Iron deficiency is associated with low haematological indices – mean corpuscular volume (MCV), mean corpuscular haemoglobin (MCH) and mean corpuscular haemoglobin concentration (MCHC). However, these are not accurate during pregnancy and only imply the diagnosis. The diagnostic test for iron deficiency is a ferritin concentration. This is not affected by pregnancy, and a concentration of $<12$ µg/L is diagnostic. **(2 marks)**

- It is widely accepted that there is an increased risk of preterm delivery and IUGR in women who are iron deficient. It is clear that those women who embark on labour with low haemoglobin do not tolerate blood loss well and therefore, from both the fetal and maternal prospectives, this needs to be corrected. **(2 marks)**

- Once the diagnosis of iron deficiency anaemia is confirmed, treatment needs to be initiated. Oral iron therapy should be commenced (ferrous sulphate: 200 mg b.d.). This should be taken with vitamin C to aid intestinal absorption. The red cell indices should be checked 2 weeks after commencing therapy. A 0.8 g/dL increase could be expected for each week of therapy. **(3 marks)**

- If there is no improvement in the haemoglobin concentration by the third trimester, compliance should be questioned. Alternative interventions may be needed. Parental iron can be given as deep muscular injection of iron sorbitol. Intravenous iron therapy preparation may also used and is associated with a greater and more rapid rise in haemoglobin concentration with fewer side effects, as compared with oral preparations. At the end of pregnancy, a blood transfusion may be required, but this is not without side effects, notably anaphylaxis. **(3 marks)**

- Folate deficiency is rare in pregnancy and a laboratory diagnosis is suggested by a macrocytic anaemia. If it is suspected, investigations should include red cell folate and vitamin B12 levels. Deficiencies during early pregnancy have been shown to increase the rate of neural tube defects in the fetus. The treatment of this rare condition should be either 5 mg oral pteroylglutamic acid daily or parenteral folate. **(4 marks)**

- In women of Asian or African origin, haemoglobinopathies may present with anaemia. If these are suspected, electrophoresis should be arranged. The management of these conditions should be in collaboration with a haematologist.    **(2 marks)**

- Chronic diseases such as tuberculosis, infections and renal failure may present with anaemia of chronic disease. This presents as a normocytic, normochromic anaemia. Investigation and treatment should be targeted to the cause.    **(2 marks)**

  *See Chapter 7.1, Anaemia.*

**15. Justify the investigation of a 39-year-old woman presenting at 34 weeks' gestation with right hypochondrial pain.**

- This woman's age should point towards the diagnosis of cholelithiasis or cholecystitis. However, it is also important to exclude other causes directly related to pregnancy such as HELLP syndrome (haemolysis, increased liver enzymes and low platelets), pre-eclampsia and acute fatty liver of pregnancy. Other possible diagnoses include hepatitis and even appendicitis. **(4 marks)**

- A full clinical history should be taken in order to evaluate whether this is a new problem presenting in pregnancy or whether it is a chronic problem with a diagnosis of gallstones already made. Relapses of cholecystitis are more common in pregnancy due to the bile stasis and increased cholesterol excretion. A history of persistent vomiting and pain should alert the clinician to the possibility of the diagnosis of acute fatty liver of pregnancy. **(6 marks)**

- Clinical signs that should be determined include the woman's temperature, as pyrexia will suggest a diagnosis of cholecystitis. Blood pressure measurement and urinary dipstick testing should be undertaken in order to exclude the diagnosis of pre-eclampsia. **(4 marks)**

- *Investigations*
    A full blood count should be obtained; a leucocytosis would indicate an infective cause for the pain and suggest cholecystitis.
    Liver function tests should be performed in order to exclude both HELLP syndrome and acute fatty liver of pregnancy.
    An ultrasound scan of the liver and bile duct should be arranged to identify whether gallstones are present; however, the absence of gallstones on the scan should not exclude the diagnosis, as up to one-third of gallstones will not be apparent on an ultrasound scan. **(6 marks)**

*See Chapter 7.2, Abdominal pain.*

**16. A 36-year-old woman who is in her third pregnancy is referred at 30 weeks' gestation with a lump in her breast. Outline the initial investigation of this patient.**

- Breast lumps are common in pregnancy and most are benign in nature. However, the clinician must be aware of the possibility of breast cancer.                    **(2 marks)**

- A full medical history should be taken and should include a detailed history of the presenting complaint: pain, onset, discharge and bleeding. Although nipple galactorrhoea is common in pregnancy, bleeding is abnormal and merits further investigation.                    **(4 marks)**

- In the past medical history it should be ascertained whether there is any history of previous breast lumps having been investigated. A detailed family history should ascertain whether there is a family history of breast cancer.                    **(2 marks)**

- A thorough medical examination should be undertaken, with specific examination of the breasts and chest. The breasts should be inspected for symmetry; the lump should be palpated and the size, shape, consistency and fixing to underlying structures noted. The breast should be expressed and any discharge should be tested for blood.                    **(3 marks)**

- If there is a suspicion of breast cancer, the woman needs referral to a breast surgeon for further management.                    **(3 marks)**

- An ultrasound of the lump should be arranged. If the lump is solid, this increases the possibility of cancer. If cancer is suspected, either a fine-needle aspiration or excisional biopsy should be performed in order to confirm the diagnosis.                    **(3 marks)**

- If a diagnosis of breast cancer is made, staging investigations should include a chest X-ray (with adequate abdominal/pelvic screening). However, either MRI or ultrasound scanning should replace CT scanning for metastases.                    **(3 marks)**

  *See Chapter 7.3, Malignancy.*

**17. A 24-year-old woman in her first pregnancy is noted to have a 6 cm adnexal mass on a dating ultrasound scan at 8 weeks' gestation. Justify your management.**

- The increase in the use of dating scans has resulted in this problem being detected more often. However, ovarian cancer is rare in pregnancy (1 in 1000 deliveries – this equates to 1 in 20–50 ovarian masses). This woman is young and therefore the risk is low; moreover, even if a malignancy is present, 30–40 per cent of tumours will be germ-cell or epithelial tumours with low malignancy potential.                                                     **(4 marks)**

- A full history should be taken to ascertain whether there are symptoms that might suggest torsion. If these are present, a laparotomy should be undertaken.         **(2 marks)**

- The ultrasound scan will give some details of the morphology of the cyst; if it is simple in nature or if the appearances are suggestive of a dermoid, the likelihood of malignancy is very low. If the cyst is multiloculated and has solid components, the likelihood of a diagnosis of cancer is increased.                                                                        **(3 marks)**

- Further information about the cyst can be obtained from an MRI scan, which is safer in pregnancy than a CT scan. Although tumour markers such as CA125, human chorionic gonadotrophin (hCG) and aFP are useful outside of pregnancy, the specificities of these markers fall in pregnancy, as these can all be elevated. Therefore, the use of tumour markers in pregnancy is not justified.                                                              **(4 marks)**

- In the absence of symptoms suggestive of torsion, or of appearances suggestive of malignancy, a conservative approach is justified. Nevertheless, 10–15 per cent of these cysts will become symptomatic. The cysts may rupture and this complication is associated with increased risk of miscarriage.                                                        **(3 marks)**

- A further scan should be arranged at 16 weeks' gestation. If the mass has increased significantly in size, a laparotomy should be considered. The surgery should be performed through a midline incision, and peritoneal washings should be taken. Either a simple cystectomy or an oophorectomy should be performed; the contralateral ovary should be inspected. However, bilateral oophorectomy should be avoided and biopsies are of little benefit. There is no proven evidence to support the use of tocolytics postoperatively.                                                                                              **(4 marks)**

*See Chapter 7.3, Malignancy.*

**18. Justify the initiation of insulin therapy in a 26-year-old woman with gestational diabetes diagnosed at 20 weeks' gestation.**

- Most cases of gestational diabetes are diagnosed in the late second and early third trimesters. Therefore a diagnosis of gestational diabetes relatively early in the pregnancy should alert the clinician to the possibility that this woman has pre-existing non-insulin-dependent or insulin-dependent diabetes.                                    **(4 marks)**

- In the management of gestational diabetes, dietary control should be the initial strategy to try to control the blood glucose level. However, if this fails, additional treatment is required. In the non-pregnant state this could include the addition of oral hypoglycaemic agents, but these should be avoided in pregnancy because of their teratogenic nature. Therefore, during pregnancy, insulin therapy is the only choice available to control blood glucose.                                    **(4 marks)**

- Insulin should be commenced if:
    after 2 weeks of dietary manipulation there is no improvement in the blood glucose control or the fasting blood glucose is >5.8 mmol/L (fasting) or 7.8 mmol/L (post-prandial).                                    **(3 marks)**
    there is evidence of fetal macrosomia despite good control with diet; insulin therapy for this indication has been found to reduce the rate of macrosomia at delivery, from 45 per cent to 14 per cent.                                    **(3 marks)**

- The commencement of insulin therapy in pregnant women with poorly controlled diabetes has been shown to reduce:
    the perinatal mortality rate
    the unexplained stillbirth rate
    the incidence of macrosomia
    the caesarean section rate
    the incidence of shoulder dystocia
    the rate and risks of polyhydramnios.                                    **(6 marks)**

*See Chapter 7.5, Gestational diabetes.*

**19. A 34-year-old woman presents at 36 weeks in her second pregnancy. Her first pregnancy was complicated by an elective caesarean section for breech presentation. She has a blood pressure of 140/90 mmHg and urine Dipstix shows 2+ proteinuria. Outline the management of this woman for the rest of her pregnancy.**

- The most likely diagnosis is pre-eclampsia; however, this needs to be confirmed. A full history is required to ascertain whether there are any risk factors for pre-eclampsia; these include previous or family history of pre-eclampsia and multiple pregnancy. The birth weight of the previous pregnancy should be noted, as this may indicate a past history of IUGR. The booking blood pressure should be noted, as this may indicate chronic hypertension.                                                                **(2 marks)**

- She should be admitted for both maternal and fetal assessment. Maternal assessment should include a full blood count to determine platelet count (not a good diagnostic test, but useful to monitor disease progression).

   Urea and electrolyte concentrations should be determined to assess renal function.

   Liver function tests should also be performed to exclude HELLP syndrome.

   A 24-hour urine collection should be initiated to confirm that the urinary protein is >0.3 g/24 hours. An urgent midstream urine and microscopy should be sent to exclude a UTI.                                                                                         **(5 marks)**

- A full medical examination of the woman should be undertaken, including a neurological examination of reflexes, which are brisk in pre-eclampsia. An abdominal palpation will demonstrate whether the fetus is clinically small for dates and whether there is epigastric tenderness.                                                              **(2 marks)**

- A CTG should be performed to assess immediate fetal well-being; if there are any abnormalities noted, delivery should be considered. An ultrasound scan is useful to determine fetal well-being and presentation.                                                  **(2 marks)**

- If a diagnosis of pregnancy-induced hypertension without proteinuria is made, the women can be monitored in the community with regular blood pressure checks and urine testing. This does not require any further intervention unless the clinical situation changes, as there is no evidence that anti-hypertensive therapy improves the outcome for the mother or fetus.                                                                       **(2 marks)**

- If a diagnosis of chronic hypertension is made, the woman may need anti-hypertensive therapy. Possible therapeutic agents include labetolol, nifedipine and methyldopa. Intensive blood pressure monitoring will be required in the community/hospital. Delivery should be considered at 38 weeks' gestation.                                          **(2 marks)**

• A diagnosis of pre-eclampsia should merit delivery. However, the previous caesarean section complicates the clinical situation. A vaginal examination should be performed to assess the cervix for induction of labour. If an artificial rupture of the membranes is possible, this should be considered after counselling with regard to the risks of uterine rupture and the risks of failure. The risk of uterine rupture with induction of labour without the use of prostaglandins is double (1.6 per cent) that of spontaneous labour (0.8 per cent). If the cervix is less favourable and would require prostaglandin priming initially, induction still can be considered; however, the complication rate is further increased and the woman should be counselled appropriately. The final option in this situation is of a repeat caesarean section for the patient.            **(5 marks)**

*See Chapter 7.6, Pre-eclampsia and non-proteinuric pregnancy-induced hypertension, and Chapter 26, Management after previous caesarean section.*

**20. Illustrate, using examples of medications prescribed for respiratory and neurological disease, how drugs and pregnancy may influence one another.**

- Pregnancy has a marked effect on pharmacokinetics. The absorption, distribution, metabolism and elimination of drugs may be increased, decreased or stay the same. The absorption of drugs from the gut may be increased by longer transit times and higher gastric pH levels. Enhanced skin and pulmonary perfusion may also increase the absorption of topical and inhaled drugs. These effects are rarely of clinical significance. Gastric emptying is usually significantly delayed during labour and this, combined with vomiting, may mean that oral drugs are poorly absorbed. **(2 marks)**

- Steroids, anti-epileptic drugs and anticholinesterases may need to be given parenterally during labour to avoid the problem of poor absorption. The volume of distribution is increased by the raised body water and fat content found in pregnancy, and this may necessitate higher starting and maintenance doses. For this reason, an increase in the dose of anticholinesterase drugs or in the frequency with which they are given is often needed for the treatment of myasthenia gravis during pregnancy. **(2 marks)**

- Postnatally, the dose may need to be changed to pre-pregnancy levels soon after delivery to prevent toxicity. Reduced albumin levels (mostly dilutional) may result in increased unbound (active) fractions, potentially leading to toxicity. This is of particular concern for anti-epileptic drugs that demonstrate >50 per cent protein binding (e.g. phenytoin and phenobarbitone). This also makes serum levels potentially misleading when used as a guide for dosing schedules, as these usually reflect 'total' drug levels rather than free 'active' drug levels. However, the significant increase in glomerular filtration rate enhances the renal elimination of many drugs and this may counterbalance any effect of reduced protein binding. Indeed, some neurologists consider that routine testing of serum levels of anti-epileptic drugs during pregnancy is unnecessary and potentially misleading. Pregnancy has a variable effect on the hepatic metabolism of prescribed drugs and this may also influence the final clinical effect of a particular dose. **(4 marks)**

- All drugs, except insulin and heparin, cross the placental barrier, reach the fetus and can have a variety of effects, including miscarriage, teratogenicity and altered fetoplacental physiology. There may be neonatal effects and longer-term problems of developmental delay and behavioural disturbance. The risk of childhood malignancies may be raised by in-utero exposure to certain anti-epileptic drugs, including phenytoin and carbamazepine. The timing of the fetal exposure is often critical to the detrimental effects the drug might have. **(4 marks)**

- Anti-epileptic drugs illustrate the risks of teratogenicity, with an approximate two–three-fold increase in the risks of neural tube defects, cardiac and genitourinary anomalies and the 'fetal anticonvulsant syndrome' following exposure during the first trimester. **(2 marks)**

- Steroids have been implicated in an increase in the incidence of cleft lip and palate, and aminoglycosides are known to be ototoxic to the fetus. Trimethoprim is a folate antagonist and is usually avoided in the first trimester due to theoretical risks of potentiating neural tube defects. **(2 marks)**

- Fetal physiology may be adversely affected by drug exposure. Anti-epileptic drugs and isoniazid (used in tuberculosis) are vitamin K antagonists and predispose to haemorrhagic disease of the newborn. Steroids may affect fetal blood pressure and cause neonatal adrenal suppression. Sulphonamides may displace protein-bound bilirubin and predispose to kernicterus. **(2 marks)**

- Finally, most drugs also reach breast milk, albeit often in very small amounts. For those drugs reaching milk in higher quantities, neonatal surveillance may be required. For example, if women using high doses of anticholinesterases breastfeed, cholinergic crisis in the newborn may result. **(2 marks)**

*See Chapter 8, Medication in pregnancy.*

## 21. Debate the use of nuchal translucency screening versus serum screening as methods of identifying pregnancies at risk of Down's syndrome.

- Both nuchal translucency (NT) and serum screening have been introduced into routine clinical practice as methods of identifying pregnancies at risk of Down's syndrome. However, neither screening method fulfils all the World Health Organization criteria for a good screening test. Both have significant benefits and deficits.    **(2 marks)**

- Both screening tests require the pregnancy to be accurately dated.    **(2 marks)**

- One of the main benefits of NT screening is the timing of the test, which can be performed between 12 and 14 weeks' gestation. This may provide early reassurance for women in high-risk groups, such as those who have previously delivered an affected baby. Nuchal translucency screening also allows women the option of a medical termination of pregnancy if invasive tests indicate an abnormal karyotype. It also facilitates early detection of associated lesions such as cardiac abnormalities.    **(4 marks)**

- The early timing of NT screening conveys disadvantages, in addition to advantages. In a proportion of the pregnancies in which it is performed, chromosomally abnormal fetuses would have spontaneously aborted by the second trimester, thus reducing the grief and anxiety produced by the decision to screen and terminate.    **(2 marks)**

- Other disadvantages of NT screening include:
    it may be an unacceptable test to the woman as she may be required to have a transvaginal ultrasound scan (TVUS) performed;
    the wide-scale introduction of NT as a screening test has cost and manpower implications that may make it cost ineffective; this includes the necessity for chorionic villus sampling to be readily available;
    there are problems with the reproducibility of the ultrasound measurements of NT screening, which are subject to observer error.    **(3 marks)**

- The biochemical serum screening tests have the advantage of being robust and reproducible, without operator error or variability. Serum screening is also widely available and potentially does not require a personally invasive test.    **(3 marks)**

- In addition to being performed at a later gestation, the disadvantages of serum screening include:
    a detection rate which is lower than that of early NT screening
    it cannot be reliably performed in multiple pregnancies, and it is altered by obesity, diabetes and ethnicity.    **(2 marks)**

- Preliminary data show that NT screening in combination with serum screening may have the highest sensitivity and specificity for the detection of Down's syndrome. However, a combination-screening programme may be difficult to achieve because of costs.

**(2 marks)**

*See Chapter 10.1, Biochemical screening.*

**22. Discuss the aims of the mid-trimester anomaly ultrasound scan, using examples of neural tube, abdominal wall and renal abnormalities.**

- The mid-trimester anomaly scan serves as a screening test for major structural abnormalities. If a lethal abnormality is detected, this may allow (after appropriate counselling) termination of the pregnancy, thus reducing the perinatal mortality rate. If termination is not accepted, the anomaly scan may also allow parents to prepare themselves psychologically for the delivery of an abnormal baby.  **(3 marks)**

- If a non-lethal abnormality is detected, in-utero therapy may be initiated to improve the prognosis at birth. Early detection will allow parental discussion with the relevant specialists with regard to prognosis and treatment.  **(3 marks)**

- The mid-trimester anomaly scan may identify 'soft markers', which do not convey disability in themselves, but which increase the likelihood of karyotypic abnormalities. These soft markers include renal pelviceal dilatation, echogenic foci and choroid plexus cysts.  **(3 marks)**

- All pregnant women should be offered the mid-trimester anomaly scan to identify these structural abnormalities, as 95 per cent of abnormalities occur in pregnancies with no prior risk factors. That said, the mid-trimester anomaly scan can be very reassuring to those mothers at particular risk of an abnormality, such as women with diabetes mellitus, a history of drug taking or a family history of a structural anomaly.  **(3 marks)**

- The scan should be carried out between 18 and 20 weeks' gestation, when the detection rate is greatest. However, it should be appreciated that certain abnormalities such as cardiac lesions require the alteration of the scan timing to 22–24 weeks to improve the positive predictive value of the test.  **(2 marks)**

- Neural tube defects have the highest detection rate of the major structural abnormalities, with anencephaly being 100 per cent. The detection of open spinal defects is 89 per cent, which is greater than with biochemical screening tests.  **(2 marks)**

- The diagnosis of an anterior abdominal wall defect allows early differentiation between gastroschisis and omphalocele. The distinction between the two conditions will determine the need for fetal karyotyping.  **(2 marks)**

- The early detection of renal agenesis allows a termination of pregnancy, as this is incompatible with life. However, the diagnosis of urethral or ureteric obstruction facilitates fetal therapy with the insertion of shunts; these protect the renal tract from damage until delivery.  **(2 marks)**

*See Chapter 10.2, Ultrasound screening.*

### 23. Discuss the indications and drawbacks of the different methods of invasive fetal testing.

- Amniocentesis is the most commonly used invasive fetal test. The major indication is for fetal karyotyping in pregnancies deemed to be at high risk on the basis of maternal age, biochemical or ultrasound screening tests or a history of a previous pregnancy in which the fetus was affected. **(2 marks)**

- Amniocentesis can be performed from 16 weeks to term. Performing the test prior to 16 weeks increases the risk of miscarriage, ruptured membranes and orthopaedic deformities, and is therefore not recommended. **(2 marks)**

- Amniocentesis is performed with a transabdominal needle and carries fetal loss rates of 0.5–1.5 per cent. The procedure is associated with an increase in neonatal morbidity from respiratory distress, orthopaedic deformities and fetal trauma. It is also associated with isoimmunization in Rhesus-negative women. **(4 marks)**

- Amniocentesis also has the advantage that it can also be used for fetal diagnosis, therapy and monitoring. **(2 marks)**

- Chorionic villus sampling is an alternative to amniocentesis. It has the similar indication of increased risk of a karyotypic abnormality on the basis of maternal age, a screening test or a previous affected fetus. However, it has the advantage that it can be performed either transabdominally or transvaginally from 10 weeks' gestation to term. **(2 marks)**

- Chorionic villus sampling has a fetal loss rate similar to that of amniocentesis and is also associated with limb deformities that correlate with gestation. One of its major disadvantages is the potential for contamination of the sample by maternal cells or the presence of placental mosaicism; this can either lead to a false-negative result or make the result difficult to interpret. **(4 marks)**

- Cordocentesis is the final method of invasive fetal testing. This involves the direct sampling of fetal blood. The procedure carries a significant increase in the mortality rate, as compared to either amniocentesis or chorionic villus sampling. The mortality rate is dependent on the indication for the procedure. Cordocentesis has the advantage of allowing diagnosis and fetal therapy at the same time. This is particularly useful in the management of Rhesus disease; anaemia can be diagnosed and treated during the same procedure. Cordocentesis also facilitates the diagnosis of fetal infections by either direct culture or polymerase chain reaction (PCR) of the fetal blood. **(4 marks)**

*See Chapter 10.3, Invasive prenatal diagnosis.*

**24. Discuss the management of a woman whose fetus is noted to have an abdominal wall defect when scanned at 20 weeks' gestation.**

- The woman should have a second scan in a tertiary centre so that it can be determined whether this defect represents a gastroschisis or an omphalocele.    **(2 marks)**

- Insertion of the umbilical cord into the sac confirms the diagnosis of an omphalocele. If this is the case, the woman and her partner should be informed and counselled that the anomaly carries a 30 per cent risk of a chromosomal abnormality. Invasive prenatal testing should be offered. There is a 10 per cent risk of associated structural abnormalities, which should be excluded with high-resolution ultrasound. The woman should be informed that if the karyotype is normal, the prognosis is good. She should also be informed that there is an overall 75 per cent survival rate; fetal morbidity includes prematurity, gastrointestinal obstruction and short gut.    **(5 marks)**

- A normal umbilical cord insertion into the abdominal wall will confirm the diagnosis of a gastroschisis. This is associated with a chromosomal abnormality rate of <1 per cent. However, this rate increases if there are associated structural abnormalities and this may necessitate counselling with regard to an invasive fetal test. The parents should be informed that the overall mortality rate is 10 per cent, and that this is because of premature delivery and ischaemic bowel.    **(5 marks)**

- Both of these conditions require similar antenatal management if the pregnancies are continued. The parents will need to be introduced to the paediatric surgeons so that the prognosis and operative details can be discussed. Serial scans should be arranged for the fetus, as both omphalocele and gastroschisis are associated with reduced fetal growth and increased liquor volume. There is no evidence that early delivery protects the fetus from the effects of amniotic fluid, and therefore vaginal delivery should be the aim unless there are other obstetric indications for a caesarean section.    **(4 marks)**

- The delivery should be conducted in a unit that has paediatric surgical facilities. At the time of delivery, the fetus requires careful handling and is placed into a protective sterile bag. The parents should be made aware that 85 per cent of defects might be closed during a primary operation. However, the other 15 per cent may require the insertion of a silastic silo to allow the defect to be closed in multiple operations.    **(4 marks)**

*See Chapter 10.4, Management of fetal anomalies.*

**25. Discuss the management of a 27-year-old woman who presents at an antenatal booking clinic having had a stillbirth at 27 weeks' gestation in her last pregnancy.**

- A detailed medical history needs to be obtained.

- The previous pregnancy notes should be reviewed, along with the results of any investigations, including fetal karyotype and post-mortem results.    **(4 marks)**

- The review of the history and of the previous records should determine whether there was any recurrent or non-recurrent cause for the pregnancy loss.    **(2 marks)**

- Recurrent causes include:
  maternal conditions such as a history of pre-eclampsia, an inherited or acquired thrombophilia or alpha-thalassaemia; each of these conditions has a significant recurrence risk
  fetal conditions include karyotypic abnormalities, such as those associated with a balanced parental translocation.    **(4 marks)**

- The identification of a recurrent cause may provide an indication for further investigation or treatment.
  If the woman has a history of pre-eclampsia, there are data to suggest that the administration of low-dose aspirin will reduce the risk of pre-eclampsia and consequent preterm delivery and stillbirth. The maternal blood pressure and urine need to be monitored closely, with serial assessments of fetal growth.
  The patient should be advised that if a thrombophilia or APS has been detected, the treatment with aspirin and heparin may improve the pregnancy outcome.
  A previous history of a fetal congenital or chromosomal abnormality may provide an indication for screening or invasive fetal testing, after appropriate counselling.
    **(3 marks)**

- The patient should be counselled that if there was no identifiable cause for the loss, the recurrence rate is low. However, the fetus remains at increased risk of IUGR and premature delivery. This will necessitate additional assessments of fetal growth throughout pregnancy.    **(4 marks)**

- The caregiver should be alert to the fact that the maternal psychological well-being may deteriorate through the pregnancy and that extra reassurance (including serial assessments of fetal well-being) may be required.    **(3 marks)**

*See Chapter 11, Previous history of fetal loss.*

## 26. Discuss the prognosis and management of a twin pregnancy complicated by fetal demise.

- Early-pregnancy loss of a twin is common, and occurs in approximately 30 per cent of twin pregnancies. Early fetal loss is associated with a good outcome for the surviving twin, even after expulsion of the dead twin. A fetus papyraceous needs to be registered as a stillbirth.                                                        **(2 marks)**

- Death of a twin occurs after the twentieth week of pregnancy in approximately 5–6.5 per cent of twin pregnancies.                                                        **(1 mark)**

- The chorionicity of the pregnancy is the major prognostic indictor for the surviving twin.
                                                        **(2 marks)**

- Monochorionic twins have distinct vascular connection between them, therefore any event that affects one of the twins can be transmitted to the other. This may occur through chemical mediators or pressure changes within the circulatory systems. Therefore, the co-twin has 25 per cent chance of fetal death. There is also a high risk of fetal neurological morbidity with cerebral palsy, cerebral infarcts and hydrocephalus.
                                                        **(3 marks)**

- The management of the death of a monochorionic twin needs careful counselling and fetal surveillance. Maternal causes for the fetal death need to be excluded and, if identified, the delivery may need to be expedited. If there is no maternal cause found, then the pregnancy can be continued on the understanding that the risk of fetal brain damage is high.                                                        **(3 marks)**

- Weekly scans should be arranged to examine for gross brain damage. If there is evidence of damage, fetocide should be offered. If the brain remains normal, intensive fetal monitoring is mandatory and postnatal MRI should be arranged.                   **(3 marks)**

- It is very uncommon for dichorionic diamniotic twins to have any vascular connections, and therefore the main risk for the surviving twin is prematurity due to either spontaneous or iatrogenic delivery. The management of the death of a dichorionic twin depends on both the gestational age and the maternal condition, as the fetus is at a low risk of an adverse intrauterine event. Maternal causes for the death should be sought and, if identified, delivery should be expedited. With a gestational age of less than 34 weeks, steroids should be administered and conservative management adopted. If the fetus is more than 34 weeks' gestation, there are few additional benefits for continuing the pregnancy; labour should be induced unless there are obstetric indications for a caesarean section.                                                        **(4 marks)**

- Conservative management of either group is associated with a risk of disseminated intravascular coagulation. Therefore this should be monitored with clotting studies; fibrinogen levels are the most sensitive indicator. **(2 marks)**

*See Chapter 12, Multiple pregnancy.*

**27. Describe the management of a pregnancy in which the mother has had a viral illness and has been demonstrated to have an acute cytomegalovirus infection.**

- Cytomegalovirus is a DNA virus that is specific for human cells only. It causes an influenza-like illness with fever, headache and sore throat and occasionally with a transient rash. It is not highly infectious but is transmitted, and sero-positivity in pregnant women is in some way dictated by socioeconomic class (high socioeconomic class 45 per cent susceptible; low socioeconomic class 15 per cent susceptible). Patients are investigated by obtaining a blood sample after a viral illness and identifying CMV IgM. However, anti-CMV IgM may persist for up to 16 weeks following a primary infection, and detection of the IgM in the first trimester may represent an infection that has occurred before conception. The diagnosis is more certain if sero-conversion after an index illness is noted.                                                      **(3 marks)**

- Cytomegalovirus infection in utero is associated with a spectrum of fetal and neonatal disease. Ultrasound findings include fetal growth restriction, microcephaly and cerebral calcification. In order of frequency these are:
    thrombocytopenia – 80 per cent
    hepatosplenomegaly – 70 per cent
    growth restriction – 40 per cent
    microcephaly – 40 per cent.                                                       **(2 marks)**

- The principal method of perinatal transmission is transplacental.        **(2 marks)**

- Transplacental transmission can occur after primary or reactivation infection. Reactivation infection is rare, occurring in between 0.5 and 1 per cent of immune women, and between 0 and 1 per cent of infected infants may have clinically apparent disease.                                                                 **(2 marks)**

- Of the susceptible individuals, 1–4 per cent have primary infection and there is an approximately 40 per cent transmission rate to the fetus. Of these, 10–15 per cent will be infected and have clinically apparent disease, of which 90 per cent will develop sequelae. Of those individuals who are apparently asymptomatic on ultrasound scan, 5–10 per cent will develop sequelae.                                                          **(3 marks)**

- Of those infected, 90 per cent have developmental delay and 60 per cent have hearing loss and neurological deficits, including abnormalities of intelligence quotient (IQ).
                                                                          **(2 marks)**

- *Management in utero.* This should include referral to a tertiary referral fetal medicine centre for a detailed ultrasound scan and detection of viral particles in amniotic fluid or fetal blood. Ultrasound may demonstrate hydrops fetalis or congenital malformations (i.e. ventriculomegaly or intracranial calcification). Also, IUGR and bowel echodensity can be noted. Isolation of CMV in amniotic fluid or fetal blood (lymphocytes) is most sensitive using PCR.                                                                          **(3 marks)**

- In fetal blood, LFTs can be performed, as can the detection of thrombocytopenia. Identification of an infected fetus often provokes the discussion of termination of pregnancy. Other than this, conservative therapy with investigation of the fetus at birth and also long-term follow-up is advised. Some individuals have used intravascular ganciclovir administered via cordocentesis to try to reduce the viral load. However, this is rather anecdotal in its use. No vaccine is available to prevent CMV and it is unlikely that epidemiologically based prevention schemes increasing immunity will be provided.                                                                          **(3 marks)**

*See Chapter 13, Fetal infections.*

**28. Describe the management of a pregnancy at 28 weeks' gestation where the symphysio-fundal height measures 24 cm.**

- Symphysio-fundal height measurements in pregnancy (increasingly customized) form a screening test for the detection of IUGR. This type of screening will only identify a baby that is small for gestation – a heterogeneous group comprising those babies that fail to achieve their growth potential (i.e. true IUGR) and those that are constitutionally small. It is babies with IUGR that are at increased risk of stillbirth, birth hypoxia, neonatal complications and impaired neurodevelopment. There is also evidence that cardio-vascular risk factors and metabolic abnormalities such as type II diabetes will be increased and track into adult life.

  A complete history should be taken and full clinical examination performed. Physical examination of the abdomen by inspection and palpation detects as few as 30 per cent small-for-gestational-age fetuses. Studies have shown that it has a sensitivity and specificity of between 27 and 88 per cent. Serial measurements may improve these figures. The use of customized fetal height charts improves the accuracy of this test.

  **(5 marks)**

- Ultrasound management of the fetus involves the exclusion of congenital abnormalities (many of which are small for gestation). Abdominal circumference (AC) and estimated fetal weight (EFW) are the most accurate diagnostic measurements to predict small for gestational age. In high-risk women, AC at less than the 10th centile has sensitivities of between 72.9 and 94 per cent and specificities of 50.6–83.8 per cent in predicting babies that are less than the 10th centile. Serial measurements enhance the accuracy of diagnosis of IUGR, and a $\Delta$AC of less than 1 standard deviation (SD) over 14 days is again indicative of impaired fetal growth. Other sorts of monitoring of fetal well-being should also be performed including:
  umbilical artery Doppler velocimetry
  liquor volume estimation.
  Biophysical profiling in ultrasound has not been shown to improve prognosis in RCTs.

  **(6 marks)**

- Once IUGR is identified, a pregnancy of high risk has been detected. In the preterm situation, maternal betamethasone should be administered to mature fetal pulmonary surfactant production and also to reduce the risk of intraventricular haemorrhage at birth. There is also some evidence that this transiently improves umbilical artery Doppler velocimetry measurements.

  **(4 marks)**

- The timing of delivery is important and no conclusive factors have been identified. Serial measurements of umbilical artery Doppler velocimetry are useful and, when absent end-diastolic flow is noted, there is some debate as to whether immediate delivery is optimal (GRIT Study). However, long-term follow-up of this group indicates that morbidity is less if the fetus is immediately delivered. A combination of umbilical artery Doppler measurements, non-stressed cardiotocographs (CTGs) – after 28 weeks' gestation – and liquor volume is used to decide on the mode of delivery and gestation at delivery. For potentially compromised babies, when delivery is required preterm, there will be a high rate of caesarean section. The place of delivery is important, and such babies should be delivered in tertiary referral neonatal units.                          **(5 marks)**

*See Chapter 14, Tests of fetal well-being, and Chapter 15, Fetal growth restriction.*

**29. Describe the management of a fetus that had a 20-week scan and that has been identified as having hydrops fetalis.**

- The woman should be referred to a tertiary referral fetal medicine centre. A full history and examination should be performed. This will give some information about whether or not the mother is Rhesus negative and has alloimmunization and about whether she has had a previous viral illness. There will also be some information to be gleaned regarding previous history of genetic abnormalities or indeed consanguinity. Special factors are important: for instance, in Chinese races the risk of alpha-thalassaemia is higher than in Caucasians in the UK.                                                              **(4 marks)**

- A detailed ultrasound scan should be performed to exclude congenital abnormalities. In particular, abnormalities of the fetal heart should be excluded and normal cardiac rate and rhythm identified.

  The diagnosis of fetal hydrops is made when there is fluid noted on ultrasound examination in two body cavities in the presence of fetal skin oedema.        **(4 marks)**

- Doppler ultrasound to assess the middle cerebral arteries is of use and the systolic peak velocity using Doppler in these arteries may be found and may give an indirect measurement of the risk of fetal anaemia. Maternal blood samples should be taken to note maternal blood group and the presence or absence of antibodies. Haemoglobin electrophoresis and bloods should be sent for virology to look for IgM antibodies to CMV, toxoplasmosis and human parvovirus B19.                                        **(4 marks)**

- Often, cordocentesis is recommended so the following investigations can be performed:
  karyotyping
  formal haemoglobin concentration and, if necessary, transfusion
  viral titres (IgM antibodies) and, if necessary, a formal viral DNA fragment by PCR
  LFTs
  storage of DNA for subsequent molecular diagnosis.                              **(4 marks)**

- The overall prognosis for a fetus in which there is no fetal anaemia is 50 per cent mortality. It is extremely important that a detailed post-mortem examination be performed for such individuals to provide additional information for the parents. For fetuses in which there is maternal alloimmunization or fetal anaemia secondary to human parvovirus infection, with serial intrauterine transfusion, the prognosis is very good, with survival >90 per cent.                                              **(4 marks)**

  *See Chapter 17, Fetal hydrops.*

**30. Discuss how you would manage a woman who is in her first pregnancy at 41 weeks' gestation and who has declined vaginal examination and induction of labour.**

- Approximately between 5 and 15 per cent of all pregnancies are post-term (>294 days). There is a plethora of information indicating that early dating ultrasound scanning significantly reduces this percentage, to approximately 6 per cent.    **(1 mark)**

- Not all babies of a prolonged pregnancy have post-maturity. It is thus the role of the obstetrician to try to identify babies at risk.

  Perinatal mortality, especially stillbirth rate, is relatively low at 40 weeks (0.86 per thousand) but increases to 2.12 per thousand at 43 weeks – an approximately three-fold increase. Similarly, neonatal mortality rates also increase during this period. It is likely that the risks of post-term pregnancy increase because of:
  meconium staining of the amniotic fluid and potential meconium aspiration syndrome
  intrapartum hypoxaemia and fetal acidosis
  fetal acidosis
  birth trauma and shoulder dystocia.    **(4 marks)**

- Prospective studies comparing routine induction of labour at 41 weeks' gestation compared to antenatal surveillance and spontaneous onset of labour have demonstrated that induction at 41 completed weeks of pregnancy will reduce perinatal morbidity and mortality and also lead to a reduction in caesarean section rate.    **(4 marks)**

- In women that opt for 'natural' onset of labour, some form of antenatal surveillance is necessary. The midwife or obstetrician needs to remain ever vigilant regarding the development of maternal disease such as pre-eclampsia. Prolonged pregnancy is a common indication of fetal assessment in terms of trying to identify fetal compromise. Fetal assessment using non-stressed CTG has been advocated as a relatively easy and non-invasive test. However, many series have indicated that this investigation can be falsely normal in up to 8 per cent of subjects with poor outcome. There have been no RCTs showing the benefit of this form of monitoring in this group.

  Several centres have indicated that amniotic fluid volume as an ultrasonic measure of maximum pool depth may give an indication of fetal compromise. While there is an association between oligohydramnios and increased risk in a post-term pregnancy, the degree of risk has not been defined accurately. It is maximum pool depth as an estimate of liquor volume that appears to be the most sensitive measure of fetal compromise at this gestation.

  This may be enhanced (although the evidence for this is shaky) by combining it with a formal ultrasound biophysical profile. Certainly, in the largest studies, a reduced perinatal mortality of 4.6 per thousand in the series of post-term pregnancies was reported using this technique.

Doppler velocimetry of the umbilical artery may have a role in fetal surveillance. In a small sample of post-term pregnancies, it was found that the umbilical artery Doppler pulsatility index did not change significantly. The absence of end-diastolic flow was used as a predictor of fetal compromise in that the fetus became distressed in the first stage of labour. In combination with amniotic fluid volume estimation, the predictive index was 100 per cent.    **(5 marks)**

- However, within this is the view that there is improved maternal choice. This comes from representative groups in the community, such as the National Childbirth Trust (NCT) and the Association for Improvements in Maternity Services (AIMS), and also the recommendations of the House of Commons Select Committee. Certainly, women at 41 completed weeks' gestation should be offered vaginal examination to sweep the membranes, and a RCT indicated that this led to an increased rate of spontaneous labour without risks.    **(2 marks)**

- Induction of labour after 41 weeks is not associated with any major disadvantage, reduces the small risk of perinatal death in women with normal pregnancies, and may result in a small reduction in caesarean section rate in these women. There is a difference between prolonged pregnancy and post-maturity, the latter indicating a pathological process. The use of surveillance may aid the detection of abnormality in these apparently normal but at-risk fetuses. However, obstetricians and pregnant women should be aware of the poor quality of evidence to support the use of all available methods of fetal surveillance commonly offered to women with prolonged pregnancy. Whether management based on epidemiological evidence of the Cochrane Centre database would be acceptable to women is unknown, and should perhaps be the subject of future research. Data examination of meta-analysis with special redress to large, prospective, multicentre trials indicates that induction of labour at 41 completed weeks was not harmful, and discussion regarding induction of labour should probably take place at this time. The need for confirmation of the correct gestation of pregnancy in terms of early ultrasound dating (between 9 and 12 weeks' gestation) cannot be over-emphasized.    **(4 marks)**

*See Chapter 19, Prolonged pregnancy.*

**31. A woman presents at 26 weeks with ruptured membranes; she is not contracting. Describe your management.**

- A full history must be taken documenting the potential duration of membrane rupture and the events surrounding this.    **(1 mark)**

- Investigation of the potential causes of the preterm pre-labour rupture of membranes should include the following.

  Swabs for infection, taken by a single sterile speculum examination. The speculum examination will also confirm the diagnosis of ruptured membranes. A digital examination must be avoided.

  Culture and sensitivity investigations performed on a midstream urine specimen to investigate for a UTI.

  Care clinical examination to assess the potential diagnoses of abruption and chorioamnionitis (maternal temperature, pulse rate, abdominal palpation).    **(3 marks)**

- Fetal assessment should be with particular reference to the difficulties of interpretation of CTG in the very preterm baby; at 26 weeks' gestation most practitioners would advocate this as a medium for fetal assessment. An ultrasound scan should be performed to determine presentation, growth and remaining liquor volume. Assessment of fetal breathing is also useful, as this is often absent with chorioamnionitis.    **(2 marks)**

- Maternal investigations include a full blood count – the white cell count (WCC) is particularly important (WCC goes up after steroid administration and remains high for 48 hours) – and the level of C-reactive protein (CRP).    **(1 mark)**

- The woman should be advised regarding the potential for preterm labour and the likely neonatal outcomes (a neonatologist should be involved).    **(1 mark)**

- Treatment to improve neonatal outcome includes steroid administration, antibiotics (erythromycin) and in-utero transfer if neonatal intensive care is unavailable. Tocolytics are of value only to facilitate transfer and possibly to allow steroid administration (although in this scenario tocolytics are rarely effective).    **(4 marks)**

- If labour does not occur within 48 hours, a concise plan for monitoring of the pregnancy should include some reference to where the patient will be managed (inpatient versus outpatient). If outpatient care is advocated, the maternal temperature must be taken regularly, and signs of bleeding, uterine activity, tenderness, 'flu-like symptoms, reduced fetal movements or offensive vaginal discharge reported.    **(2 marks)**

- Surveillance for chorioamnionitis should include WCC at least weekly, with CRP estimation as a possible adjunct. Maternal temperature should be measured at least twice daily.                                                                                    **(2 marks)**

- Fetal surveillance should incorporate CTG; this can demonstrate rising fetal heart rate (often the first sign of chorioamnionitis). The optimal frequency of CTG is debatable, but should probably be at least daily if inpatient care is advocated. Ultrasound assessment of fetal well-being can be valuable; again, the optimal frequency is debatable. Growth should be assessed fortnightly.                                                          **(2 marks)**

- The gestation at which delivery should be advised is contentious, although some data from RCTs suggest that induction at 34–36 weeks is the best policy. The use of repeated steroid doses if labour does not occur after 2 weeks is also controversial (there is increasing anxiety regarding repeat courses).                                             **(2 marks)**
*See Chapter 22, Pre-labour rupture of membranes.*

**32. A 30-year-old primigravida attends the antenatal clinic 3 days after her expected date of delivery. The pregnancy has been problem free. How would you advise this woman?**

- Dates should ideally be calculated from a first trimester ultrasound rather than from the last menstrual period, as this is more reliable. **(2 marks)**

- Pregnancy prolonged after 41 completed weeks is associated with a progressive rise in perinatal mortality and morbidity. **(2 marks)**

- None of the commonly used tests of fetal well-being (e.g. kick chart, CTG, amniotic fluid measurements, Doppler velocimetry) reliably predicts fetal compromise in this situation. **(3 marks)**

- Induction of labour should be offered after 41 weeks and delivery should be accomplished by 42 weeks. **(2 marks)**

- A policy of routine induction after 41 weeks is clearly supported by evidence that:
  perinatal mortality and morbidity are reduced
  the instrumental delivery and caesarean section rates are reduced. **(3 marks)**

- Most women favour induction of labour. However, if the offer of induction is declined, a strategy of increased monitoring should be offered, including weekly assessment of amniotic fluid index and twice-weekly CTG. Induction should be strongly recommended if there is a reduction in liquor volume. Any reduction in fetal movements should be reported urgently. **(3 marks)**

- At 41 weeks, a membrane sweep should be offered, with appropriate counselling regarding discomfort and 'post-sweep' bleeding. **(3 marks)**

- The woman should receive information regarding the process of induction of labour. **(2 marks)**

*See Chapter 25, Induction of labour.*

## 33. Critically comment on the management of slow progress during the active phase of the first stage of spontaneous labour in a multiparous woman.

- Slow progress is recognized by a poor rate of cervical dilatation. An underlying aetiology is infrequently determined. **(2 marks)**

- The management of poor progress may include a combination of:
  artificial rupture of membranes
  maternal rehydration
  augmentation with intravenous Syntocinon
  the provision of adequate analgesia. **(4 marks)**

- There is no evidence that augmentation in the first stage of labour alters outcome when compared with non-intervention, though labours are generally shorter. Maternal satisfaction scores are higher when labour is shortened. **(1 mark)**

- Many women will respond to other measures such as hydration and the presence of the continuous support of a professional. These should be tried prior to oxytocin administration. **(1 mark)**

- Augmentation with Syntocinon in a multigravida is associated with a higher risk of uterine rupture. It should only be considered when there has been a full assessment of the progress by a senior doctor. **(2 marks)**

- This must include assessment of:
  the fetal size
  the findings on vaginal examination (dilatation, position, descent, moulding)
  the contraction frequency
  fetal and maternal condition. **(4 marks)**

- Where there is evidence of obstruction, augmentation should not occur and delivery by caesarean section should be considered. **(2 marks)**

- If Syntocinon is used, a plan must be made for re-assessment. Continuous electronic fetal monitoring should be used. **(2 marks)**

- The mother's views about the management strategy are important. **(2 marks)**
  *See Chapter 27, Poor progress in labour.*

**34. You are called to a fetal bradycardia that has occurred 10 minutes after the siting of an epidural. Discuss your management.**

- It is important to remember that epidural analgesia is a common cause of fetal bradycardia. Bradycardia can occur in the absence of demonstrable reduction in maternal blood pressure. **(2 marks)**

- Strategies should be directed towards improving placental blood supply by correcting:
  maternal hypovolaemia and/or hypotension
  maternal positioning to avoid aorto-caval compression
  intravenous fluids when appropriate
  vasoconstrictors such as ephedrine for lower limb vasodilatation secondary to epidural analgesia
  if Syntocinon is running, this should be stopped and only restarted once the fetal condition is satisfactory. **(4 marks)**

- Maternal oxygen therapy should not be used for more than a short period of time unless there is a documented low maternal oxygen saturation. **(1 mark)**

- A full assessment of the clinical picture should be performed, including determination of the obstetric risk factors and progress in labour. The development of any risk factors in labour should be noted (meconium/bleeding/poor progress/fever etc.). **(4 marks)**

- The previous CTG should be examined and a decision made with regard to the tolerance of the fetus, taking into account the clinical picture prior to the bradycardia. **(2 marks)**

- If the fetal bradycardia is not resolving, the rule of threes should be followed (3 minutes to assess, 3 minutes to remedy the cause, 3 minutes to plan delivery and 3 minutes to transfer and expedite delivery). **(3 marks)**

- If the bradycardia resolves and the CTG becomes normal and was normal prior to the bradycardia, scalp pH sampling is not necessary. **(2 marks)**

- If the bradycardia resolves but the CTG prior to this was abnormal, a scalp sample should be performed after a period of 10 minutes. **(2 marks)**
  *See Chapter 29, Fetal compromise in the first stage of labour.*

**35. What precautions should be taken at a caesarean section for a placenta praevia in order to minimize maternal blood loss? If excess blood loss occurred, what would your management plan be?**

- The following precautions should be taken.

   The presence of a senior surgeon and anaesthetist should be ensured.    **(2 marks)**

   The operation should be performed as an elective procedure rather than as an emergency (where possible).    **(1 mark)**

   The advantages/disadvantages of a regional versus general anaesthetic should be considered.    **(1 mark)**

   Uterine relaxants such as halothane should be avoided.    **(1 mark)**

   Prophylactic oxytocin therapy (bolus and infusion) should be administered following delivery.    **(1 mark)**

   Spontaneous placental separation should be allowed before any attempts at controlled cord traction.    **(1 mark)**

   If spontaneous placental separation does not occur, the aim is to separate the placenta from the upper segment of the uterus first.    **(1 mark)**

- The management options if severe haemorrhage ensues include the following.

   Administration of oxytocin: bolus (10 IU) and infusion (40 IU in 500 mL 0.9% saline over 4 hours).    **(2 marks)**

   Prostaglandin therapy: administered intramuscularly, intramyometrially or by a vaginal pessary.    **(2 marks)**

   Surgical methods of attaining haemostasis: over-sewing major bleeding points, uterine compression sutures, ligation of internal iliac arteries, caesarean hysterectomy, embolization.    **(4 marks)**

   The protocol for severe postpartum haemorrhage should be instigated, including liaison with a haematologist regarding fresh frozen plasma/cryoprecipitate.    **(2 marks)**

   Serious problems occur when the decision to perform a hysterectomy is unduly delayed.    **(2 marks)**

*See Chapter 31, Caesarean section.*

**36. You are asked to assess an abnormal cardiotocogram in a woman at term in her first pregnancy. The cervix is fully dilated, but she has an effective epidural and is not pushing. Describe your management.**

- Assessment of the CTG should include assessment of the baseline, variability, presence and type of decelerations. A rapid assessment should determine whether urgent delivery is required (e.g. bradycardia), and a comparison with the previous CTG should be made to determine changes in the pattern and the duration of abnormality.    **(4 marks)**

- There should be an assessment of risk for fetal compromise:
  growth restriction, pre-eclampsia, bleeding etc.
  the progress of the labour – and the use of oxytocin
  a vaginal examination should be performed to assess the feasibility of delivery.
  **(3 marks)**

- Concomitantly, steps should be taken to:
  1. improve placental blood supply:
     maternal positioning to avoid aortocaval compression
     intravenous fluids when appropriate
     vasoconstrictors such as ephedrine for lower limb vasodilatation secondary to
     epidural analgesia    **(3 marks)**
  2. improve maternal oxygenation:
     maternal oxygen therapy may be helpful if used for a short period while other
     measures are instituted    **(2 marks)**
  3. diminish uterine activity if excessive:
     decrease or stop any oxytocin infusion
     consider tocolysis (in the second stage, bolus i.v. tocolytics have been associated
     with an increase in instrumental delivery but no improvement in fetal outcome)
     **(2 marks)**
  4. consider whether a fetal scalp sample is indicated:
     if an easy assisted delivery is not possible
     the CTG is of concern; however, if the pH is normal, labour could be allowed to
     continue.    **(2 marks)**

- A decision must then be made regarding the need for urgent delivery, based upon:
  severity of the CTG abnormality and results of any secondary tests of fetal well-being
  response to above interventions to improve situation
  the 'whole picture', including obstetric risk factors, progress in labour and potential
  difficulty of an assisted delivery
  untreatable fetal complications such as abruption, cord prolapse and chorioamnionitis
  scar dehiscence.    **(4 marks)**

*See Chapter 32, Fetal compromise in the second stage of labour.*

## 37. Shoulder dystocia presents a significant risk-management problem. Outline the strategies that can be employed to minimize this risk.

- The fact that neither fetal macrosomia nor shoulder dystocia can be reliably predicted means that every member of the delivery staff should know how to deal with this complication. **(1 mark)**

*Antenatal management*
- It is recognized that most strategies to prevent shoulder dystocia are either ineffective (early induction) or lead to excessive intervention (elective caesarean section). Fetal macrosomia in the presence of diabetes represents the only condition in which shoulder dystocia is predictable (but even then there is disagreement about which estimated fetal weight should stimulate a recommendation for caesarean section). **(2 marks)**

- A plan should be made for women who have had a previous shoulder dystocia antenatally. Where there was significant neonatal or maternal trauma, the mother should be counselled carefully about the next delivery. **(1 mark)**

*Training and guidelines*
- There should be a clear guideline as to the management of shoulder dystocia, with which all obstetric and midwifery staff should be familiar.
  The guideline should outline the circumstances in which shoulder dystocia is more likely, to ensure appropriate alerting of senior staff for delivery:
    fetal macrosomia
    maternal diabetes
    slow progress in labour
    previous shoulder dystocia. **(5 marks)**

- All staff should have the opportunity to rehearse strategies to manage shoulder dystocia on a regular basis (annually). **(1 mark)**

- Obstetric drills can be helpful to identify training issues. **(1 mark)**

*Management in labour*
- The presence of known risk factors, particularly two or more, should trigger advance preparations to deal with or avoid the situation, before it actually arises.
    Senior input should be sought before attempting instrumental vaginal delivery where there is an increased risk of shoulder dystocia.
    If instrumental delivery is undertaken, consideration should be given as to the best place for this (i.e. in the operating theatre).
    When a severe shoulder dystocia occurs, the appropriate people should be summoned: the most senior available obstetrician, the duty anaesthetist and neonatal staff.
  **(4 marks)**

*Documentation*
- Accurate documentation is vital. This should include:
  timing (especially from delivery of the head to delivery of the body)
  manoeuvres
  resuscitation
  perineal trauma.                                          **(4 marks)**

- Parental debriefing should occur at an appropriate time.   **(1 mark)**
  *See Chapter 33, Shoulder dystocia.*

**38. A woman consults you at her booking visit in her second pregnancy at 12 weeks as she wishes to discuss delivery. She sustained a third-degree tear after a lift-out forceps in her first pregnancy. How would you advise her?**

- A full history should be taken. This should include careful questioning regarding:
  short-term problems after delivery
  long-term symptoms of faecal/flatus incontinence
  problems with sexual intercourse
  the performance of additional investigations, for example endoanal ultrasound
  the necessity for any other interventions.                      **(5 marks)**

- A careful review of the notes should be undertaken to assess the extent of the trauma and the events surrounding delivery.                      **(3 marks)**

- Following this, the woman may fall into one of several categories.
  1. If she was and is asymptotic, counselling should cover the risks of further sphincter damage (approximately 4 per cent) and strategies to avoid this, including recommendations regarding:
     epidural (increased risk)
     ventouse if she needs instrumental delivery
     episiotomy – only if indicated at delivery (2 marks should be deducted for recommending elective episiotomy).
     A recommendation for vaginal delivery should be made and discussed with the woman. Transient incontinence after a first delivery carries a risk of worsening of symptoms after subsequent delivery in 20 per cent of cases.      **(5 marks)**
  2. If the woman has continued to be symptomatic, counselling should explain that a vaginal delivery is associated with a risk of worsening of symptoms.
     If a decision is made to proceed with a vaginal delivery, a risk-avoidance strategy should be adopted. Many women will choose caesarean section.      **(4 marks)**
  3. If the woman has undergone a secondary anal sphincter repair, it should be recommended that she be delivered by caesarean section.      **(3 marks)**

*See Chapter 36, Perineal trauma.*

**39. A premature infant is delivered at 28 weeks' gestation. Outline the important principles involved in maximizing outcome in the first few minutes.**

- The resuscitator should be aware of the increased risk of respiratory distress syndrome in premature deliveries. This is due to surfactant deficiency, leading to non-compliant lungs, with difficulty maintaining a functional residual capacity, alveolar collapse, cardiovascular compromise and fatigue due to increased work of breathing.    **(2 marks)**

- Important resuscitation principles include the following.

    Preparation of appropriate equipment and personnel: it is worth considering the availability of replacement surfactant. Early use of surfactant results in better outcome from respiratory distress syndrome than late, 'rescue' therapy.    **(2 marks)**

    Good communication: the parents should be aware of the likely course of events, and kept informed of progress.    **(2 marks)**

    A relevant clinical history, including confirmation of gestation and exclusion of other potential complicating factors such as infection.    **(2 marks)**

    Premature infants loose heat rapidly, which increases the risk of adverse events such as hypoglycaemia, acidosis and further surfactant reduction. The infant needs to be kept warm from early on.    **(2 marks)**

    A rapid assessment of the clinical condition should be performed.    **(1 mark)**

    Not all infants at 28 weeks require intubation. Assessment of the respiratory effort, heart rate, colour and activity takes seconds and can determine how the resuscitation should proceed. An infant making good respiratory effort, with a good heart rate above 100 bpm and good perfusion, may simply need monitoring and warmth before transfer to the neonatal unit.    **(2 marks)**

    In contrast, an infant with poor respiratory effort, cyanosis and poor heart rate needs additional help. The airway should be properly positioned and cleared of excessive secretions. The lungs will be stiff and poorly aerated; hence there may be the need for five initial rescue breaths. These are prolonged, forceful breaths to establish a functional residual capacity, thus improving lung compliance. Subsequent respiratory support will be guided by the infant's response. It may be wise to consider early elective intubation. This ensures a secure airway and enables much more effective delivery of breaths.    **(3 marks)**

    Standard teaching is to use 100 per cent oxygen. However, this may be detrimental to the premature lung; hence early monitoring and careful assessment to reduce the risks of hyperoxia are important. Equally, the premature lung is very delicate, and the combination of barotrauma and volutrauma can cause a lot of damage. Early administration of surfactant may help to reduce this.    **(2 marks)**

    Once the infant appears stable, all lines, tubes etc. should be secured and the infant transferred to a neonatal unit for ongoing support.    **(2 marks)**

*See Chapter 38, Neonatal resuscitation.*

## 40. How does knowledge of the physiological adaptations the newborn infant undergoes influence your approach to resuscitation in neonates?

- All resuscitation situations rely on the ABC (airways, breathing and circulation) approach, and the newborn infant is no different. However, there are important physiological changes the infant undergoes between existence in the uterine environment and independent life, which, if upset, may lead to difficulties.    **(2 marks)**

- The first consideration relates to the changes affecting the airway and respiration. The vast majority of neonatal (and indeed paediatric) arrests are primarily respiratory in origin.    **(2 marks)**

- Surfactant plays a major role in lung compliance in the newborn. Surfactant production does not become fully matured until late in the third trimester, and then it is not distributed within the alveoli until the infant takes its first few breaths of air. Surfactant production can be affected by a number of factors, including prematurity, hypoxia and cold temperature.    **(4 marks)**

- The mechanism leading to the passage of meconium and the effect of meconium on the fetal/neonatal airway should be explained.    **(2 marks)**

- The role of rescue breaths, clearing of meconium and surfactant therapy should be discussed.    **(2 marks)**

- The changes in the neonatal cardiovascular system include closure of the ductus venosus, the foramen ovale and the ductus arteriosus.    **(2 marks)**

- Pulmonary vascular pressures change with the first few breaths; the fall in pulmonary pressures coincides with a release of vasodilators into the pulmonary circulation.    **(2 marks)**

- Adequate oxygenation is necessary in order to allow these changes to occur and to prevent persistence of the fetal circulation.    **(2 marks)**

- Temperature management is important, as cold stress can be a major cause of morbidity in the newborn.    **(2 marks)**

*See Chapter 38, Neonatal resuscitation.*

**41. The routine newborn examination is an important screening tool in the first few days of life. Discuss.**

- It is standard practice to perform a neonatal examination within the first few days of life in the UK.                                                                          **(1 mark)**

- The role of the newborn examination as a screening test should be discussed with particular reference to the following.

  The potential benefits of reassurance. The examination gives parents reassurance that health professionals are taking an interest. It can help to reassure them that everything is fine with their child at that moment. It can also be a useful opportunity to discuss any concerns, such as feeding, as well as to give general health advice, such as about vaccinations.                              **(3 marks)**

  The alternative argument is that the examination simply gives false reassurance at an unpredictable time. It is a crude test with poor sensitivity and specificity and may simply lead to blame and recrimination when problems subsequently occur that 'should have been picked up at birth'.                                      **(3 marks)**

- Explanation to the parents should include the fact that the examination can have both false positives and false negatives, with particular reference to examples such as the following.

  Cardiac examination: cardiac murmurs are much more common in the first 24 hours of life, and significant cardiac lesions can be missed due to lack of signs in the early days.                                                                             **(2 marks)**

  'Clicky' hips: these are probably simply due to lax ligaments secondary to excessive levels of maternal hormones in the infant. It can be difficult to distinguish those hips that will settle from those that are unstable and likely to develop into dislocated hips. Also, it has been repeatedly shown that dislocated hips are missed during the newborn examination.                                           **(3 marks)**

- Strategies to improve the discriminant ability of the newborn examination include the following.

  The identification of higher risk infants, who should receive further investigation. For example, most units have developed guidelines to select babies for hip ultrasound investigation.                                                                    **(4 marks)**

  Better education and 'hands-on teaching' so that the examination is always performed correctly.                                                                           **(2 marks)**

  Better education of parents so that they understand the examination in the context of a screening test.                                                                    **(2 marks)**

*See Chapter 39, Common neonatal problems.*

**42. A 26-year-old woman has just delivered a 5.0 kg baby. As the obstetric registrar on call, you are urgently summoned to the labour suite. When you arrive in the room, the woman is shocked, the blood loss is 100 mL, and your differential diagnosis includes an inverted uterus. Detail the management of this woman.**

- Initially, the on-call consultant should be informed and asked to attend. The anaesthetist should also be called to the delivery suite, as a general anaesthetic may be indicated. The senior house officer should be present to facilitate various tasks. The most senior obstetrician present should take charge of the situation.                                **(2 marks)**

- The woman's airway should be secured and oxygen administered. Vital signs should be assessed and monitored. Intravenous access should be established and bloods taken for an urgent full blood count and cross-matching, as the woman may require an examination under anaesthetic. If the woman is clinically shocked, intravenous crystalloid should be commenced.                                **(4 marks)**

- An abdominal examination should be undertaken. A uterine fundus that is not palpable is consistent with the diagnosis of an inverted uterus. A vaginal examination should confirm uterine inversion.                                **(2 marks)**

- If the placenta remains undelivered, no attempts should be made to remove it until the uterus is replaced into its anatomical position. Removal of the placenta without re-inversion of the uterus may cause excessive haemorrhage.                                **(2 marks)**

- If analgesia is adequate, the uterus should be replaced manually. This is possible if the diagnosis is made rapidly; however, it becomes more difficult due to tissue swelling.                                **(2 marks)**

- If this is unsuccessful, the woman will require a general anaesthetic, at which time it may be possible to replace the uterus manually. However, if this fails, O'Sullivan's method, utilizing hydrostatic pressure, should be attempted. This involves filling the vagina and uterus with warm saline and obstructing the introitus so that the resultant pressure reverses the inversion.                                **(3 marks)**

- The failure of O'Sullivan's method will necessitate the patient having a laparotomy. Haultain's procedure should be performed before the uterus becomes ischaemic from obstruction of its blood supply. Traction is placed on the round ligaments and an incision is made through the muscular ring in the posterior uterine wall. Continued manual pressure on the fundus from the vagina and traction of the round ligaments will allow replacement of the uterus, and the incision is then closed.                                **(3 marks)**

- After successful re-inversion of the uterus, the placenta should be manually removed if still present. A Syntocinon infusion should be commenced to encourage uterine contraction.                                                         **(2 marks)**

*See Chapter 41, Postpartum collapse.*

## 43. Describe the management of a patient with retained placenta.

- The definition of a retained placenta is one that has not been delivered after 15 minutes (given that 90 per cent of placentas spontaneously deliver within 14 minutes). It is widely agreed that patients with retained placenta are at significantly increased risk of haemorrhage.                                                                                    **(2 marks)**

- Predisposing factors to retained placenta are:
    previously retained placenta
    multiparity
    induced or preterm labour
    history of previous instrumentation of the uterus
    placenta praevia
    leiomyomata.                                                                                    **(6 marks)**

- Placenta accreta is a particularly morbid condition associated with retained placenta and is becoming more common. The risk factors for this are:
    placental praevia
    abnormally elevated second trimester maternal serum aFP
    raised $\beta$hCG in the second trimester
    being 35 years or older.
  The risk of previous caesarean section also increases the risk of morbidly aberrant placenta.                                                                                    **(4 marks)**

- Management should include the siting of a large-bore intravenous cannula with infusion of crystalloid. Bloods should be taken for full blood count and group and save. (If there is significant haemorrhage with cardiovascular compromise, bloods should be cross-matched.) Patients should be catheterized and an anaesthetist should be informed.
  The patient should be transferred to theatre. A check should be made to ensure that the placenta is not in the cervical canal or in the vagina prior to an anaesthetic. Excessive traction and fundal pressure should be avoided – otherwise the risk of uterine inversion is increased. Prophylactic antibiotics should be given, and then a manual removal of the placenta under appropriate anaesthesia should be performed.                              **(4 marks)**

- There is some evidence that intra-umbilical oxytocic agents may be efficacious. Certainly, active management of the third stage with intramuscular Syntometrine should be undertaken.                                                                                    **(2 marks)**

- If there is continual bleeding or difficulty in removing the placenta, senior help should be obtained because of the possibility of morbidly adherent placenta and the need for caesarean section.                                                                                    **(2 marks)**

  *See Chapter 42, Postpartum haemorrhage.*

**44. A 19-year-old woman who is 8 days postnatal, having undergone an emergency caesarean section for failure to progress, is admitted with a pyrexia of 38.5 °C. Discuss the possible diagnoses and subsequent management.**

- Postpartum pyrexia is a common occurrence, with an incidence of approximately 5 per cent. The aetiology can be broadly divided into four separate categories:
  benign fever
  breast engorgement/infective mastalgia
  infection of the urogenital tract
  distant infection.                                              **(2 marks)**

- Benign fever occurs in 3 per cent of women in the early postpartum period, with resolution in the first 24 hours. This needs no specific treatment.          **(1 mark)**

- The most common cause of pyrexia postnatally is a UTI. The patient will present with dysuria, frequency and lower abdominal pain. This pain will be situated over the bladder and may radiate to the loins. A clean-catch urine specimen should be collected and Dipstix analysis may show protein and nitrates, which would indicate a UTI. The specimen should be sent for microscopy and culture. Broad-spectrum antibiotic therapy should be initiated; however, this should be altered according to the results of urine culture.                                              **(4 marks)**

- Wound infection is the next most common cause of a postpartum pyrexia. It is suggested by a history of abdominal pain located around the abdominal scar. On examination, there may be erythema and discharge from the wound. Microbiology swabs should be taken for culture and sensitivity. However, the woman should be commenced on antibiotics prior to these results being obtained. If there is a wound abscess present, this will require incision and drainage.                                              **(4 marks)**

- Endometritis is another common infection that can occur in the postnatal period. It presents with fever, rigors and an associated offensive vaginal discharge; the uterus may be palpable and tender, with the cervical os open. A vaginal swab should be taken and antibiotics commenced.                                              **(2 marks)**

- Breast engorgement/infective mastalgia will present with a history of breast pain. Examination may reveal an enlarged, erythematous breast. Anti-inflammatory drugs can be used to alleviate the pain, and antibiotics prescribed if infection is considered likely. If a breast abscess is present, it will need incision and drainage.                                              **(2 marks)**

- Distant sites of infections include postoperative chest infections, secondary to atelectasis. The patient may present with a productive cough. Examination findings include evidence of consolidation at the lung bases. Sputum should be sent for culture. Antibiotics and supportive therapy with oxygen and physiotherapy are required.

**(3 marks)**

- A pulmonary embolism may present with pyrexia and therefore any patient whose diagnosis is questioned should be investigated. This may necessitate a ventilation/perfusion (V/Q) scan and treatment with anticoagulants. **(2 marks)**

*See Chapter 43, Postpartum pyrexia.*

## 45. Discuss the possible psychiatric sequelae of pregnancy and how these might be prevented or treated.

- Disturbances in the emotional state are common in the postnatal period. Up to 80 per cent of women will experience some form of emotional alteration, which occurs most commonly between days 3 and 10 and is characterized by tearfulness, irritability and insomnia. However, unlike most mental illness, it resolves within 48 hours and responds to kindness. **(4 marks)**

- Mild postnatal depression affects 7 per cent of postnatal women. It is associated with social adversity, single status and poor support. The history is of an insidious onset of insomnia and difficultly in coping. The most effective treatment for mild depression is counselling, which is as effective as antidepressant therapy in this group of patients. **(4 marks)**

- Severe postnatal depression occurs in 3–5 per cent of all women. Most cases can be detected at the 6-week postnatal check by use of the Edinburgh postnatal score. Thirty per cent of women with this condition will present within the first 3 months after delivery. They may present with a history of early-morning wakening, altered appetite and ahedonism. The management should include explanation and reassurance. Tricyclic antidepressant therapy is effective, with results observed within 2 weeks of commencing treatment. The course should be maintained for 6 months. Both oestrogen and progesterone therapy have been advocated. The woman should be informed that in subsequent pregnancies the recurrence rate is approximately 50 per cent. **(5 marks)**

- Postpartum psychosis affects 2 in 1000 women. One-third of these women will present with an acute episode of mania; the other two-thirds will present with depression. Acute management should be aimed at sedation with neuroleptic drugs, which allows both containment and assessment. **(3 marks)**

- In cases of psychosis, a psychiatrist with an interest in postpartum psychiatric disorders should perform an assessment, which should coincide with admission to the closest mother and baby unit. The woman should be continued on an oral neuroleptic agent such as haloperidol; these drugs have extrapyramidal side effects, which can be treated with procyclidine. Lithium carbonate can be used for the mother who presents with a manic pathology. For women with severe depression, the first-line treatment is electroconvulsive therapy. The mother should be continued on treatment for at least 6 months, and advised that there is a 50 per cent recurrence rate. **(4 marks)**

*See Chapter 44, Disturbed mood.*

**46. With references to specific examples, outline the benefits and risks of breastfeeding to the mother and the newborn infant. Utilizing the same examples, also demonstrate how rates of breastfeeding can be maximized.**

- There are considerable data to support the fact that breast milk is the optimum food for babies.                                                                                  **(1 mark)**

- Evidence includes a reduction in the incidence of neonatal seizures. It has also been demonstrated that the incidence of childhood atopy and middle ear infections is reduced amongst children who have been breastfed. There is a reduction in the incidence of sudden infant death syndrome, and a lower incidence of autoimmune conditions such as juvenile-onset diabetes.                                                                      **(4 marks)**

- There are also maternal benefits of breastfeeding; these include a reduction in the incidence of ovarian epithelial cancers and of premenopausal breast cancer, as well as the financial advantages. Total breastfeeding (i.e. breastfeeding without bottle feeding) is also an effective contraceptive.                                                              **(3 marks)**

- The main risk to the baby does not come from breastfeeding itself, but from the horizontal transmission of infectious diseases. Therefore, it is suggested that women who are HIV positive should refrain from breastfeeding to prevent transmission. Similarly, women who are diagnosed as having tuberculosis and who remain untreated should refrain from breastfeeding until they are classified as non-infectious.          **(3 marks)**

- Mothers who are taking various drugs, such as senna, lithium carbonate and nalidixic acid, are advised not to breastfeed, as these agents have detrimental effects on the newborn baby.                                                                                    **(2 marks)**

- It may be appropriate to prescribe dopamine agonists to stop the production of milk in women who are advised to refrain from breastfeeding.                                      **(1 mark)**

- The maternal risks of breastfeeding result from complications such as mastalgia, which is defined as painful breasts. Simple anti-inflammatory agents provide effective relief from this problem.                                                                              **(2 marks)**

- Infective mastaglia can arise from infection with *Staphylococcus* species. The treatment of this condition is the administration of intravenous antibiotics. However, the mother should be encouraged to continue breastfeeding during this treatment.                  **(2 marks)**

- Although uncommon, breast abscesses do occur in the postnatal period. The mother should stop breastfeeding where there is evidence of pus drainage through the nipple. Once an abscess has formed, it requires surgical drainage in combination with the administration of broad-spectrum antibiotics. **(2 marks)**

  *See Chapter 45, Problems with breastfeeding.*

# GYNAECOLOGY

**47. You have delivered a baby with ambiguous genitalia. How is this problem managed?**

- The incidence of intersex conditions in the UK has been estimated at 1 in 2000. Initially it is essential that the parents have adequate psychological support, as this can be a difficult time. They should be encouraged not to register the birth or decide on a name until a diagnosis has been established. **(3 marks)**

- The decision about the sex of rearing should be made in consultation with the parents. However, it should be based on the diagnosis, appearances of the external genitalia and the chances of fertility and a fulfilling sexual relationship. **(2 marks)**

- The overall management of these cases involves a multidisciplinary team, which includes a paediatric gynaecologist, surgeon and urologist. It should also include a clinical geneticist to advise about the cause of the problem and the recurrence rate if a further pregnancy is considered. Individuals with different intersex conditions may require specific medical and surgical treatments; however, all should have access to experienced clinical psychologists and peer support via the relevant national support organizations. **(4 marks)**

- The primary investigation that needs to be performed is karyotyping from a buccal smear so that the genetic sex may be assigned. The results should be available within 48 hours and will aid gender assignment. **(1 mark)**

- The possible diagnoses should be considered next. The most common cause is congenital adrenal hyperplasia, which presents with a masculinized female at birth and may initially go undiagnosed. The diagnosis should be suspected with all cases of ambiguous genitalia. The diagnosis should be confirmed by measuring the early 17-alpha-hydroxyprogesterone levels, which will be significantly elevated. If the diagnosis is confirmed, mineralocorticoid therapy needs to be initiated immediately, as the neonate is at risk of a salt-losing crisis. **(4 marks)**

- The female neonate can also be masculinized by maternal ingestion of masculinizing drugs such as norethisterone or, rarely, through an androgen-secreting tumour. **(2 marks)**

- Partial androgen insensitivity is the most common cause of the under-masculinized male fetus. This is an X-linked disorder with a wide spectrum of clinical presentations. It is associated with an increased risk of seminomas in later life.    **(2 marks)**

- Mixed gonadal dysgenesis is another cause of the under-masculinized male, and presents with hypospadias and palpable testes in the inguinal canals. As these testes are dysgenetic, there is a 25 per cent chance of malignancy and therefore they need to be surgically removed.    **(2 marks)**

  *See Chapter 46, Normal and abnormal development of the genitalia.*

**48. An 18-year-old presents with primary amenorrhoea. How will you try to establish the cause of this from the history and examination? Discuss which investigations would be appropriate.**

- The history needs to be elicited; however, there are several specific areas in the history that may indicate the diagnosis. The most common cause of primary amenorrhoea is constitutional delay; therefore the family history is of great importance. The ages of menarche of the mother and any sisters should be determined. If these were later than normal, the patient can be reassured and informed that hereditary delay is the probable cause. A family history of polycystic ovarian syndrome (PCOS) may suggest this as a possible diagnosis, especially if the patient is overweight.    **(2 marks)**

- In the past medical history it should be noted whether there have been any significant illnesses, treatment with radiotherapy or chemotherapy, or any medications that could have damaged the ovaries or delayed puberty. Any problems at birth that may suggest a history of congenital adrenal hyperplasia should be enquired about.    **(2 marks)**

- A developmental history should be sought. This should determine the age at which the breasts and pubic hair started to develop, and whether she is still within the growth phase, as menstruation does not occur until after its onset. It should also be determined whether she is involved in sporting activities that may lead to weight-related amenorrhoea.    **(2 marks)**

- Other stresses within the family and/or at school, features that are suggestive of anorexia nervosa or the use of illicit drugs need to be determined. This is probably best achieved without the mother present.    **(2 marks)**

- During the examination, the woman's height and weight need to be determined and the body mass index calculated. Tanners' stages of secondary sexual development need to be documented. Primary amenorrhoea secondary to Turner's syndrome may be evident from the examination, with the presence of widely spaced nipples, webbed neck and wide carrying angle. Hirsutism and acne are suggestive of polycystic ovaries. The presence of good breast development and sparse pubic hair in a tall girl could suggest androgen insensitivity. Vaginal examination is not indicated; however, inspection of the external genitalia to check vaginal patency and exclude an imperforate hymen with cryptomenorrhoea is useful.    **(5 marks)**

- The initial investigations will be determined by the history and examination. Karyotype determination may reveal Turner's syndrome (45X) or androgen insensitivity (46XY).    **(2 marks)**

- It is important to measure follicle-stimulating hormone (FSH)/luteinizing hormone (LH) levels, as they may indicate several diagnoses. Raised FSH/LH levels would suggest gonadal dysgenesis; low FSH/LH levels would suggest hypogonadotrophic hypogonadism, and a raised LH/FSH ratio would be suggestive of PCOS. Prolactin concentrations should be determined, as hyperprolactinaemia can present as a readily treatable cause of primary amenorrhoea. **(4 marks)**

- An ultrasound should be arranged to exclude Rokitansky's syndrome: congenital absence of the uterus and upper vagina. It can also be used to exclude cryptomenorrhoea. **(1 mark)**

  *See Chapter 48, Menarche and adolescent gynaecology.*

## 49. Briefly discuss the recent advances and possible future developments in contraception.

- Natural methods of contraception have become popular over the last decade with women who are trying to space their families. The most popular of the available methods is the Persona™. This measures the concentrations of urinary hormones and, after several cycles, can indicate the unsafe time in the month based on the urinary LH surge. The Persona™ is associated with a method failure rate of 6.2 per hundred woman-years (HWY).                                                                                    **(3 marks)**

- Barrier methods of contraception have increased in their popularity with the advent of human immunodeficiency virus (HIV) and acquired immunodeficiency syndrome (AIDS). Condoms are now available in a variety of sizes and shapes. The advent of the spermicide nonoxinol '9' has enhanced the effectiveness of this method of contraception. The published failure rate is in the region of 3–23 per HWY. The female condom has also been introduced; however, it has not gained much popularity. Its reported failure rate is similar to that of the male condom, at 5–21 per HWY.                              **(3 marks)**

- The oral contraceptive pill has advanced significantly in recent years. One of the major advances is the introduction of lower dose oestrogen and progesterone concentrations, which has increased the safety profile with regard to venous thrombosis. Developments have also included the introduction of the alternative progestogens desogestrel and gestodene. These have a higher affinity for the progesterone receptor and thus increased effectiveness at inhibiting ovulation and giving good cycle control with low doses. However, they are associated with an increased risk of venous thrombosis.    **(4 marks)**

- Progesterone-only methods of contraception have also advanced over the last few years as their safety with respect to venous thrombosis has been shown to be better than that of combined methods. They are available as oral and other systemic preparations. They include Depo-Provera®, Implanon® and the Mirena® intrauterine device. The failure rates for these methods are 0.5 per HWY, 0.5 per HWY and 0.2 per HWY respectively.

  **(3 marks)**

- There have also been advances in intrauterine contraceptive device (IUCD) technology. Over the last 20 years, they have evolved from inert plastic frames to frames that now contain copper and, more recently, progestogen. All of these innovations have reduced the failure rate. More recently, a frameless copper device (GyneFix®) has been developed to overcome the common side effects of the framed devices.                           **(3 marks)**

- Methods of sterilization have also improved, with more laparoscopic sterilizations being performed. This has increased day case surgery and reduced the need for hospital gynaecology beds. Hysteroscopic sterilization has also been introduced.        **(1 mark)**

- Postcoital contraception has been introduced, initially with the PC4 and now with Levonelle®-2. These methods have an 80–90 per cent success rate of preventing pregnancy.                                                    **(2 marks)**

- Future contraception may include vaccines or oral male preparations.      **(1 mark)**
  *See Chapter 50, Contraception, sterilization and termination of pregnancy.*

**50. A 49-year-old woman presents at the gynaecology clinic. On examination, she is found to have a 16-week-sized fibroid uterus. Discuss the management of this patient.**

- Initially, a full medical history needs to be taken, including the symptoms that she may be experiencing. The patient may complain of menorrhagia and dysmenorrhoea. She may have the symptoms of anaemia, such as lethargy, tiredness and dizziness. She may also complain of pressure symptoms secondary to the actual size of the uterus, and this may also trigger urinary symptoms. These urinary symptoms may be cyclical as the uterus enlarges with the onset of menstruation.                                    **(4 marks)**

- Basic investigations should include a full blood count. This may demonstrate anaemia or polycythaemia secondary to the fibroid uterus. An ultrasound should be arranged to determine the size, position and number of the fibroids contained within the uterus. Magnetic resonance imaging (MRI) scans might also be used to determine anatomical sites. However most units would not offer this as a first-line investigation due to the expense.                                    **(2 marks)**

- Any irregularity in the menstrual pattern should prompt an endometrial assessment; this can be either with a pipelle or hysteroscopy.                                    **(2 marks)**

- As the risk of malignancy is low, treatment options include conservative management if the patient is asymptomatic and there is no evidence of anaemia. However, if the patient is symptomatic and requires treatment, the available options should be discussed.                                    **(2 marks)**

- There is no evidence that non-steroidal anti-inflammatory drugs (NSAIDs) decrease the size of fibroids, although they can be useful for the control of dysmenorrhoea. There is no evidence that the oral contraceptive pill causes enlargement of fibroids; indeed, long-term use may be protective. Although, there are no randomized, controlled trials (RCTs) demonstrating the beneficial effects of the oral contraceptive pill in the reduction of menstrual blood loss, several small studies have shown a benefit; therefore it is not an unreasonable modality if there are no other contraindications. However, in view of the patient's age, it may not be the most appropriate option.                                    **(2 marks)**

- Progestogens have not been shown to reduce the size of fibroids and thus their use should only be for symptomatic menorrhagia associated with anovulation. Although, the Mirena® coil has been shown to reduce the size of fibroids in case reports, it has a higher spontaneous expulsion rate. In a similar way to oral progestogens, it can be used for the treatment of symptomatic menorrhagia and is not an unreasonable choice in a 49 year old to relieve her symptoms until the onset of the menopause. Treatment with gonadotrophin releasing hormone (GnRH) agonists induces amenorrhoea and shrinkage of fibroids. After cessation of therapy, there is rapid re-growth. However, combined with add-back hormone replacement therapy (HRT), this is an option until the menopause.

    **(4 marks)**

- The classical surgical intervention that could be offered is the hysterectomy. This could either be total or sub-total, depending on the size and position of the fibroids and the cervical smear history. The use of GnRH analogues prior to hysterectomy has been shown to reduce intraoperative blood loss, and may allow a vaginal hysterectomy as opposed to an abdominal procedure.

    **(2 marks)**

- Myomectomy is another recognized treatment; however, there is always a small risk of having to proceed to hysterectomy and women should be made aware of this. A more recent approach is the use of interventional radiology to embolize the fibroids. This is a new technique that has not been fully evaluated.

    **(2 marks)**

    *See Chapter 51.2, Uterine fibroids and menorrhagia.*

## 51. How should menorrhagia be investigated and treated?

- A full medical history should be taken. A menstrual history should be obtained, which should determine the length of cycle and the number of days that the patient bleeds during her period. The severity of the bleeding pattern should be gauged; however, actual blood loss is highly subjective, but a general impression may be gained by ascertaining how many pads or tampons a patient is using and how often these are changed. The duration of the abnormal bleeding pattern should be determined. Also, a detailed account of current and past contraception use and smear history is required.

  **(4 marks)**

- A full blood count should be performed and iron therapy given if the patient has iron deficiency anaemia. Thyroid function tests should only be performed if there are suggestive features present. No other endocrine investigations are necessary in uncomplicated cases of menorrhagia. The uterine cavity should initially be investigated using transvaginal ultrasound, and the diagnosis of uterine polyps can be enhanced with the use of hydrosonography. An endometrial biopsy should only be considered for a woman who has persistent menorrhagia despite treatment. There is no evidence that a dilatation and curettage gives any additional diagnostic information over and above an outpatient hysteroscopy with endometrial biopsy.       **(6 marks)**

- The initial treatment of menorrhagia should be with tranexamic acid and mefenamic acid. These treatments can be used in combination and are effective at reducing heavy menstrual blood loss. If there are no contraindications to the oral contraceptive pill, this is a cheap and highly effective method of reducing menstrual blood loss.    **(4 marks)**

- Although the use of luteal phase norethisterone is common, it has no proven benefit in the treatment of menorrhagia other than that associated with anovulation and therefore should be avoided. However, both progestogen-releasing and continuous long-acting progestogens are effective for the treatment of menorrhagia and should be considered.

  **(2 marks)**

- If uterine polyps or small submucous fibroids have been detected on ultrasound scan or hysteroscopy, removal may be beneficial. The latest Royal College of Obstetricians and Gynaecologists (RCOG) guideline recommends that this be performed hysteroscopically.

  **(2 marks)**

- Although hysterectomy is a widespread and highly effective treatment for menorrhagia, there are now recognized effective alternatives. These include endometrial ablation techniques, which are becoming increasingly popular with both women and gynaecologists alike.       **(2 marks)**

*See Chapter 51.3, Heavy and irregular menstruation.*

**52. A 16-year-old girl presents to the gynaecology clinic as she is suffering from painful periods that are not relieved by aspirin. Discuss the logical steps in the diagnostic process and the treatment options available.**

- Severe dysmenorrhoea in young women is rarely due to any underlying abnormality. One exception is pain secondary to congenital abnormalities that are associated with menstrual flow obstruction. However, a detailed history of the pain should be sought. This should include the onset, duration and type of pain. If it is constitutional, the pain will classically be a temporary cramping lower abdominal pain that may radiate to the lower back and thighs. It is often associated with gastrointestinal and neurological symptoms. The pain should be temporary and relieved by the cessation of menstruation. Any other associated symptoms should be noted and a detailed menstrual history should also be taken.                                                                      **(3 marks)**

- Abdominal examination will normally be unremarkable. Vaginal examination is not indicated in a girl who is virgo intacta; however, it may be reassuring in one who is sexually active.                                                                                          **(2 marks)**

- In any teenage girl for whom treatment has been initiated and failed, an ultrasound scan should be arranged to exclude any uterine abnormality.                        **(2 marks)**

- The diagnosis of primary dysmenorrhoea should be explained to the patient. Reassurance should be given and the physiological process underlying the situation should be explained. In many cases this is all that is required.                              **(2 marks)**

- As the pain is thought to be due to the release of prostaglandins, NSAIDs should be prescribed. Response rate ratios generally favour naproxen and ibuprofen, aspirin having the lowest response rate ratio. Therefore the patient should be given a trial of an alternative NSAID. If the dysmenorrhoea is associated with menorrhagia, tranexamic acid may be added to reduce menstrual flow.                                      **(3 marks)**

- The oral contraceptive is an effective treatment of primary dysmenorrhoea. It also has the added advantage of reducing menstrual loss and is an effective contraceptive if this is desired. Surgical procedures such as presacral neurectomy are not considered appropriate for this condition because of their complication rates.                  **(3 marks)**

- Endometriosis is a rare cause of dysmenorrhoea in adolescent girls. It would present with pain prior to the onset of menstruation. Vaginal examination, if appropriate, could reveal pain and uterosacral nodules. An ultrasound scan should be performed, as endometriosis is associated with female genital tract abnormalities and needs to be excluded. A laparoscopy should only be performed if treatment has previously failed and would reveal typical nodules and scarring. The treatment should initially include continuous progestogens or the combined oral contraceptive pill (COCP).                    **(3 marks)**

- If the patient is sexually active, pelvic inflammatory disease (PID) is a possible diagnosis. Vaginal examination would reveal cervical excitation, and cervical swabs should be taken. The treatment is with antibiotics: doxycycline, cephalexin and metronidazole.

**(2 marks)**

*See Chapter 51.4, Dysmenorrhoea.*

## 53. What is the clinical presentation of endometriosis? How would you manage infertility associated with endometriosis?

- Endometriosis can present in a variety of ways. However, the most common presenting symptom is pelvic pain between the periods, which affects between 40 and 60 per cent of women with symptomatic disease. Heavy and irregular periods that are associated with secondary dysmenorrhoea are another common presenting symptom. This pain classically occurs prior to the onset of menstruation, gets worse with menstruation and is only relieved after menstruation. **(3 marks)**

- Dyspareunia is another common presenting symptom that affects between 30 and 40 per cent of women with symptomatic disease. Normally this is deep dyspareunia as opposed to superficial; however, it may occasionally present in an episiotomy scar after childbirth. **(2 marks)**

- Dyspareunia may also present as a generalized discomfort and the feeling of distension. Vaginal or abdominal examination may reveal a pelvic or ovarian mass. **(2 marks)**

- Between 15 and 60 per cent of women who present with subfertility, although asymptomatic, will have endometriosis present on diagnostic laparoscopy. **(2 marks)**

- Rarely, endometriosis can present with cyclical haematuria, rectal bleeding or haemoptysis. **(1 mark)**

- The management of endometriosis with regard to infertility still remains controversial. At the present time, there are no clear data to suggest which of the options affords the best outcome in terms of pregnancy rate. The options include no treatment, medical treatment with or without surgery, and surgical treatment by laparoscopy or laparotomy. **(2 marks)**

- Current evidence suggests that medical treatment has no benefit over no treatment in terms of the crude pregnancy rate. **(2 marks)**

- Laparoscopic removal of endometriotic deposits in moderate and severe endometriosis has been shown to significantly increase the pregnancy rate. However, the role for surgery in mild or minimal disease is less clear-cut, with many studies only demonstrating a minimal increase in fecundity. Therefore, surgical treatment for mild disease must be balanced with the procedure-related risks. The addition of postoperative medical therapies has not been shown to improve the pregnancy rate over surgery alone and therefore cannot be advocated. Whether preoperative medical treatment has any role still remains to be elucidated. **(3 marks)**

- In-vitro fertilization (IVF) is an effective method of treatment for endometriosis-related infertility, whatever the stage of the disease. It has also been shown that intrauterine insemination in conjunction with ovarian stimulation is an effective treatment in women with mild or moderate disease. **(3 marks)**

*See Chapter 51.5, Endometriosis and gonadotrophin releasing hormone analogues.*

## 54. Discuss the diagnosis and management options of premenstrual tension.

- Premenstrual tension is common, with 80–90 per cent of women complaining of at least one symptom. However, only 5 per cent of women suffer from true premenstrual syndrome (PMS). There are three main criteria that define PMS: (i) it must occur in the luteal phase of the cycle, (ii) it must have a major impact on life events, and (iii) it must disappear with menstruation.                                            **(4 marks)**

- It is also important to consider the family and social history. Many women complain of PMS at the time of stressful life events. There is an association with a previous history of child abuse, dysfunctional families, high-pressure jobs and alcohol misuse.    **(2 marks)**

- Examination and investigations will be normal.                              **(2 marks)**

- There are many non-hormonal treatments that have been suggested for PMS. Alteration in diet has been advocated, although there are no trials to support this. Several studies have examined the effect of the addition of trace elements such as magnesium and calcium; however, there is no clear evidence that these treatments are of benefit. Other studies have examined the addition of vitamin B6 to the diet and some have shown a positive effect on symptom relief, although, long term, high-dose use appears to be associated with peripheral neuropathy. Evening primrose oil has not been shown to have any effect on PMS, although it does relieve the associated breast tenderness. Diuretics have also been used with little effect. The serotonin uptake inhibitor fluoxetine has been demonstrated in RCTs to have a beneficial effect on the symptoms of PMS and therefore is a useful treatment. Mefenamic acid has also been shown to improve symptoms.
                                                                        **(6 marks)**

- There is little evidence for the use of oral progestogens in the management of PMS. However, Depo-Provera®, which causes ovarian suppression, may be of benefit, but requires further evaluation. Evidence regarding the COCP in the management of PMS is still unclear, as many studies show differing results. However, a trial of combined oral contraceptive therapy may be beneficial. Several studies have shown a clear benefit for the use of danazol; however, its side effects limit long-term use.       **(4 marks)**

- There are reports in the literature of the efficacy of oophorectomy; however it is not recommended for the management of PMS unless the problem is very severe, has been confirmed by prospective assessment and there has been genuine failure of conservative therapies. It should not be considered unless supported by a trial of ovarian suppression with a GnRH agonist.                                              **(2 marks)**

*See Chapter 51.7, Premenstrual syndrome.*

## 55. Discuss the management of tubal disease as a cause of infertility.

- Tubal factor is responsible for 40 per cent of female fertility cases. The commonest cause of tubal damage is PID. *Chlamydia* infection is responsible for most cases of PID in the Western world. Prevention or early treatment of this condition can potentially prevent subsequent tubal damage and reduce the risk of infertility. Identification of high-risk groups enables the initiation of screening or public education programmes.    **(2 marks)**

- For well-established cases, the treatment depends on the extent of tubal damage, the patient's age, her ovulatory status and the male factor. The treatment modalities available for tubal factor infertility are tubal surgery and IVF. In the presence of anovulation and/or poor sperm quality, IVF is a realistic and better option to consider. In the absence of these two factors, the pros and cons of the two treatment modalities should be weighed in each case individually.    **(2 marks)**

- The advantages of tubal surgery are that, if successful, it offers the patient the chance of having more than one pregnancy if desired, it has a normal risk of multiple pregnancy, no risk of ovarian hyperstimulation syndrome (OHSS), and lower cost. However, it is a major procedure that requires general anaesthesia and therefore has potential risks. Furthermore, even in expert hands, success rates are poor, which suggests that tubal surgery should be carried out in specialized centres and in highly selected cases.
    **(4 marks)**

- The feasibility of the procedure depends on the extent and site of tubal damage. Both open microsurgery and laparoscopic surgery offer similar results with regard to intrauterine and ectopic pregnancy rates. Peritubal adhesions also affect the outcome. The lysis of flimsy adhesions offers better pregnancy rates compared to that of dense adhesions. Transcervical canalization of a proximal tubal occlusion offers better pregnancy rates than surgery. The procedure can be carried out hysteroscopically or under image guidance.    **(4 marks)**

- In-vitro fertilization treatment offers better cumulative pregnancy rates than tubal surgery. However, the cost per pregnancy is significantly higher. The rate of multiple pregnancy, especially of the high-order type, has been significantly higher with IVF, which increases the perinatal mortality and morbidity as well as the cost to the National Health Service (NHS). Recent guidance to restrict the number of embryos transferred to only two has reduced the higher order multiple pregnancy rates associated with IVF.
    **(4 marks)**

- In-vitro fertilization is also associated with the risk of OHSS, which is a potentially fatal condition. The emotional involvement and stress associated with IVF treatment and the ethical issues surrounding this modality of treatment may favour tubal surgery in certain cases.    **(2 marks)**

- The patient's age should be considered when evaluating the treatment options. The fact that it will take up to 2 years after successful tubal surgery for the outcome of the procedures to become clear means that younger patients are better suited to this treatment. On the other hand, patients over the age of 40 have a significantly reduced chance of success with IVF, which may strengthen the argument in favour of tubal surgery in such cases.                                                  **(2 marks)**

*See Chapter 52.2, Female infertility.*

### 56. Semen analysis is a laboratory investigation with inherently low sensitivity and specificity. Discuss.

- Sperm quality is subject to a large biological variation and can be affected by external factors as well as by the general health of the individual. Such variability has not allowed the creation of reliable normal ranges and cut-off points in order to quantify the chances of pregnancy in a given situation. **(3 marks)**

- Semen analysis should be carried out twice if the first result is obviously abnormal or borderline according to the reference ranges adopted. **(2 marks)**

- The World Health Organization (WHO), having examined a large number of semen samples across the world, has produced reference ranges and refrained from using the terminology 'normal ranges'. These ranges can be useful in identifying potential male factor infertility. **(3 marks)**

- The WHO reference ranges and their methodology should be applied, with emphasis on the quality control, both internal and external, given the subjectivity and the nature of the test. If centres choose to adopt different methodology, they should report their reference ranges and validate them for the relevant population and should satisfy the requesting clinician with regard to their internal and external quality control procedures. **(4 marks)**

- The variations of the reports amongst different centres and laboratories have led to the repeat of many tests, and it is only prudent that GPs use the same laboratory as that used by the centre to which the couple will be referred to avoid unnecessary waste of time and resources. **(3 marks)**

- The establishment of a regional centre should be encouraged to solve such problems. An agreed protocol should be shared amongst the primary, secondary and tertiary care centres in order to streamline infertility investigations generally and to provide patients with reliable information about their fertility potential, particularly where there is a large overlap between normal and abnormal results. **(5 marks)**

*See Chapter 52.3, Male infertility.*

**57. The latest advances in assisted reproduction technology have led to a significant increase in multiple pregnancy rates, especially high-order ones. This is an iatrogenic problem that should be dealt with effectively. Discuss.**

- A previously held belief was that the pregnancy rate correlated with the number of embryos transferred. This resulted in an increase in high-order multiple pregnancy rates.                                                                 **(2 marks)**

- High-order multiple pregnancy is associated with significantly high perinatal mortality and morbidity, mainly due to prematurity. Furthermore, any rise in the multiple pregnancy rates increases pressure on neonatal units and can be detrimental. **(3 marks)**

- In the UK, the Human Fertilisation and Embryology Authority (HFEA) was created to control and govern the practice of assisted reproduction from the ethical point of view. Increasing the neonatal mortality and morbidity deliberately is an unsafe medical practice and is ethically unacceptable. Therefore, it was stipulated that the number of embryos transferred should not exceed three. Many countries do not have any governing bodies such as the HFEA, and the practice of multiple embryo transfer is still prevalent in these countries.                                                              **(4 marks)**

- Other infertility treatment modalities such as ovulation induction with or without intrauterine insemination can also lead to unacceptably high multiple pregnancy rates. Because of these observations, the British Fertility Society recommends cancellation of ovulation induction cycles where more than three mature follicles are recruited. An alternative is to convert such cycles to IVF.                                    **(3 marks)**

- Ovulation induction and intrauterine insemination using the partner's semen are practices that do not require a licence from the HFEA. However, ignoring current good practice guidelines is not acceptable.                                            **(2 marks)**

- Even with the transfer of three embryos, the multiple pregnancy rates are still unacceptably high. Recent evidence shows that optional transfer of two or three embryos does not affect the pregnancy rates, but the latter is associated with significantly increased multiple pregnancy rates – hence the recent trend to transfer only two embryos in most cases, a practice that has gained popularity across the UK and Europe.                        **(3 marks)**

- Although the practice of reducing the number of embryos transferred is still voluntary, transferring three embryos has become unpopular and unacceptable practice in the UK except under special circumstances. However, many struggle to define such special circumstances. Growing research into blastocyst culture and subsequent transfer may allow one-embryo transfer, which will reduce the multiple pregnancy rates to the naturally expected levels.                                                          **(3 marks)**

*See Chapter 52.4, Assisted reproduction.*

## 58. Discuss the clinical manifestations, diagnosis and management of polycystic ovarian syndrome.

- Polycystic ovarian syndrome refers to the presence of polycystic ovaries in women with a particular cluster of symptoms, which includes amenorrhoea, oligomenorrhoea, hirsutism, anovulation and other signs of androgen excess such as acne and crown pattern baldness. Polycystic ovaries may be diagnosed in the absence of any clinical manifestations.                                                                    **(3 marks)**

- Ultrasound is the most reliable test for the diagnosis of polycystic ovaries. The diagnostic criterion of at least ten discrete follicles of <10 mm diameter, usually peripherally arranged around an enlarged, hyperechogenic central stroma, is considered diagnostic.
                                                                                          **(2 marks)**

- Biochemical tests such as the LH:FSH ratio and elevation in androgens are unhelpful in defining the syndrome, as the levels are inconsistently elevated. Other limitations of the biochemical diagnosis of PCOS include the variable and imprecise nature of the assays and the dynamic nature of hormonal steroidal release from the ovaries.    **(2 marks)**

- The initial management of diagnosed PCOS depends on the clinical presentation. Initially, an explanation of the condition should be undertaken.                 **(2 marks)**

- If fertility is the presenting problem or is a priority for the woman, it is important that the patient optimizes her health before embarking on specific fertility therapy. The principle of the management of anovulatory infertility in women with PCOS is to induce regular unifollicular ovulation whilst minimizing the risk of multiple pregnancy and OHSS. Ovulation induction strategies should begin with simple measures.     **(2 marks)**

- Specific and effective approaches to induce ovulation in women with PCOS include weight loss in women with an elevated body mass index, clomiphene citrate and gonadotrophin therapy. Laparoscopic ovarian drilling is also an effective treatment for anovulation, but is more interventional and requires general anaesthesia. The use of metformin and other drugs that affect insulin resistance in the management of PCOS still requires further evidence.                                                                    **(5 marks)**

- Patients not wishing to conceive may still require treatment to address the androgenic symptoms of PCOS. Anti-androgens such as cyproterone acetate and spironolactone are of value. The oral contraceptive pill will also reduce the level of free androgen; however, it is important to choose an oral contraceptive with a low progestogenic effect.
                                                                                          **(2 marks)**

- Women should be advised of the long-term risks of PCOS, including an increase in the risk of ovarian and endometrial cancers. There is also an increased risk of pregnancy-induced hypertension and gestational diabetes in women with PCOS who do conceive. **(2 marks)**

*See Chapter 53, Polycystic ovarian syndrome.*

## 59. Critically appraise the treatment options available for hirsutism.

- The main principle of the treatment of hirsutism is to interrupt the excess production of androgens or remove the hair either temporarily of permanently.                                    **(1 mark)**

- Cosmetic measures are available; these include shaving, which, despite women's concerns, does not increase the rate of growth. Electrolysis is a permanent method; however, it is not funded by the NHS and courses can be expensive. These methods can be utilized in combination with medical therapies, which can take up to 6 months to have an effect.                                                                                            **(3 marks)**

- Pharmacological methods broadly fall into two categories: those methods that suppress androgen production by the ovary and the adrenal gland, and those methods that reduce the effects of androgens in the skin.                                                                            **(2 marks)**

- Ovarian suppression can be achieved by several inexpensive and effective methods, including the COCP and injections of medroxyprogesterone acetate. These have the effect of suppressing LH and increasing sex hormone-binding globulin (SHBG), thus reducing androgen levels. If the COCP is used, it should be a third-generation pill as these contain progestogens with less androgenic activity. However, they are unsuitable if conception is a priority or the patient has associated hypertension or diabetes. The other method of ovarian suppression is with the use of gonadotrophin releasing hormone (GnRH) analogues. These are more acceptable if given with low-dose COCP or HRT. However, they are unsuitable for long-term use, due to their effect on bone mineral density, or if conception is a priority.                                                                            **(6 marks)**

- There are several drugs that act to reduce the peripheral actions of the androgens. Cyproterone acetate is an anti-androgenic drug that reduces the effect of androgens at their target organs. It also reduces the secretion of gonadotrophins. However, it is unsafe in pregnancy because of its anti-androgen effects, and has to be taken in combination with oestrogens for ovarian suppression. There are also several side effects that may cause decreased compliance, including depression, weight gain, breast tenderness and decreased libido. It is also unsuitable if conception is a priority or there is associated hypertension.

  Spironolactone is an oral aldosterone antagonist with anti-androgenic properties. Flutamide is pure non-steroidal anti-androgen. Hepatotoxicity is an infrequent but serious side effect, and therefore liver function tests should be performed for the first few weeks. Finasteride is a 5-alpha-reductase inhibitor, which, as a result of its mode of action, is significantly teratogenic (emasculation of male fetus), and therefore effective contraception must always be used. Its use should be limited to severe cases only, under tertiary centre supervision.                                                                            **(6 marks)**

- There are also non-pharmacological methods of treatment of hirsutism. If the patient is obese, weight loss should be suggested, as this has the effect of reducing insulin resistance, increasing SHBG and thus reducing free testosterone concentrations. Surgical treatment with ovarian drilling in women with PCOS only offers a temporary reduction in the androgen concentrations and so is only useful for the treatment of infertility.

**(2 marks)**

*See Chapter 54, Hirsutism and virilism.*

**60. Discuss the various steps in the investigation of an 18-year-old student who has failed to commence menstruation. She has otherwise normal secondary sexual characteristics and no obvious abnormalities on general examination.**

- The first step is to exclude a pregnancy, and it might also be valuable to exclude hypothyroidism, which, although rare, is a readily treatable condition.     **(2 marks)**

- The next step is to confirm that there is a normal and functional outflow. It might be apparent on examination that there is absence of the uterus or an imperforate hymen, and the history might suggest cryptomenorrhoea. A progesterone challenge test using medroxyprogesterone acetate 10 mg b.d. for 5 days is useful, as, if positive, it is reliably suggestive that the problem is one of anovulation. Failure to provoke a withdrawal bleed after sequential oestrogen and progestogen is highly suggestive of a uterine or vaginal anomaly.     **(4 marks)**

- If oestrogen levels are low, measurement of the gonadotrophins will determine whether this is an ovarian or hypothalamic–pituitary axis problem.     **(2 marks)**

- In this patient, raised gonadotrophins would suggest resistant ovary syndrome or premature ovarian failure.     **(2 marks)**

- If ovarian failure is considered likely, chromosomal analysis should be performed. Mosaicism of the Y chromosome and, rarely, Turner's syndrome with a mosaic genotype, although unlikely, are possible explanations.     **(2 marks)**

- If the gonadotrophins are low or normal, serum prolactin should be measured and, if >1000 IU/L, an MRI of the head should be ordered. These findings suggest either a prolactin-producing adenoma or compression of the pituitary stalk.     **(4 marks)**

- In women who are otherwise normal apart from low or normal range gonadotrophins, the cause of amenorrhoea is hypothalamic, due to suppressed pulsatile GnRH secretion. This may be the result of stress, severe weight change, an eating disorder or excessive exercise. Such features should be apparent from a careful history.     **(4 marks)**

*See Chapter 55, Amenorrhoea and oligomenorrhoea.*

**61. A 55-year-old woman with severe hot flushes and night sweats presents in the gynaecology clinic. She had a lumpectomy and radiotherapy for breast cancer 4 years previously. Her mother is wheelchair-bound because of severe osteoporosis. Discuss the treatment options and justify your management.**

- It is important to establish the duration and severity of the symptoms and to determine how they affect her quality of life.                                                    **(2 marks)**

- Oestrogen is effective in the treatment of menopausal symptoms but it is implicated in the aetiology of breast cancer. Oestrogens stimulate breast cell lines. Oophorectomy and oestrogen withdrawal are useful in the treatment of breast cancer. A large meta-analysis has shown that prolonged HRT use is associated with a small but significant increase in the risk of breast cancer.                                                    **(4 marks)**

- This risk increases with duration of use, but there is no increased risk of dying from breast cancer. One would therefore be reluctant to prescribe HRT to patients with established breast cancer, and few patients with breast cancer have been prescribed HRT.                                                    **(3 marks)**

- The observational studies that have been published do not show an increased risk, but it is very likely that HRT was prescribed in patients who were at a low risk of recurrence. No randomized study has been published to show that HRT is safe in these circumstances, but the risk, if any, is likely to be small, and provided the patient is aware of the possible risk, it may be reasonable to prescribe HRT to relieve symptoms.
                                                    **(3 marks)**

- It would be reasonable to prescribe a progestogen such as norethisterone first, as this may well relieve the symptoms. Tibolone may also be useful, as it probably has less effect on the breast.                                                    **(2 marks)**

- The patient is obviously concerned about long-term osteoporosis. A bone density scan would be useful to determine the severity of disease and, if necessary, a selective oestrogen receptor modulator (SERM) might be appropriate.                                                    **(2 marks)**

- Discussion should take place with her breast surgeon and her oestrogen receptor status should be determined. She will require long-term treatment to prevent osteoporosis. The combination of a SERM and HRT might look attractive but has yet to be tested. She is probably too young for bisphosphonates, but they may be useful later.                **(4 marks)**

  *See Chapter 56, Menopause and hormone replacement therapy.*

**62. A 25-year-old nulliparous woman presents with 7 weeks of amenorrhoea and a positive home pregnancy test. She has experienced abdominal pain and vaginal spotting of blood for 24 hours. Discuss the differential diagnosis and investigation and briefly outline the treatments available.**

- This is a common scenario encountered by gynaecologists. There are several possible diagnoses, including:

  complete miscarriage

  incomplete miscarriage

  threatened miscarriage

  ectopic pregnancy

  non-specific bleeding from the genital tract.                                      **(4 marks)**

- A detailed medical history needs to be obtained. This should focus on whether the bleeding is associated with any abdominal pain and, if so, whether the onset of the pain was prior to or after the bleeding. Classically with an ectopic pregnancy, the pain precedes the bleeding, and visa versa in a miscarriage. The type and amount of blood loss need to be determined. If the loss is heavy with clots, this would be more suggestive of a miscarriage than an ectopic pregnancy. However, if the loss is port-wine coloured and minimal, this would suggest an ectopic gestation. Abdominal examination may reveal generalized tenderness or, if there were an ectopic gestation, this might be localized to one or other iliac fossa. In the case of an ectopic gestation, vaginal examination may reveal a closed cervix and tenderness in one iliac fossa. Vaginal examination in the case of a threatened miscarriage would reveal a closed cervix. An inevitable or incomplete miscarriage would reveal an open cervix.                                      **(4 marks)**

- A full blood count should be done to ascertain whether the haemorrhage has been significant and, if the haemoglobin is <9 g/dL, a transfusion should be considered. The blood group needs to be determined and serum should be saved so that if the haemorrhage increases or the haemoglobin decreases, blood can be transfused. Rhesus status should be ascertained as anti-D may be required if the patient requires a surgical intervention. The beta human chorionic gonadotrophin ($\beta$hCG) concentration should be determined as this may aid the diagnosis of an ectopic pregnancy. Intravenous access should be obtained and the patient should be starved, as surgery may be required.                                      **(4 marks)**

- In women having a first trimester spontaneous miscarriage, there is evidence to suggest that expectant management is an alternative to surgical evacuation. Several studies, both community and hospital based, have demonstrated high spontaneous resolution rates for incomplete and missed miscarriage. Although medical treatment with mifepristone and misoprostol is an option, it does not seem to offer any significant advantages in terms of reduced surgical intervention rates. Both drugs are also associated with significant side effects in up to 50 per cent of patients. Therefore, women with spontaneous incomplete or inevitable miscarriages in the first trimester should be counselled accordingly and offered a choice between expectant and surgical management. **(4 marks)**

- Although most ectopic pregnancies probably resolve spontaneously (70 per cent), and the trend towards earlier diagnosis may be resulting in over-treatment, the standard treatment for an ectopic gestation remains laparotomy and salpingectomy or salpingostomy. Whilst this is still the gold standard for haemodynamically compromised patients, laparoscopic procedures are becoming increasingly popular. Laparoscopy has several advantages related to hospital admission times. However, it is also associated with a higher subsequent intrauterine pregnancy rate and lower recurrent ectopic rate. Therefore it should be considered in all appropriate cases and where fully trained staff are available. There are several randomized studies confirming that medical treatment with methotrexate in selected cases of ectopic pregnancy is as effective as laparoscopic treatment. **(4 marks)**

*See Chapter 57, Problems in early pregnancy.*

**63. A 32-year-old woman complaining of recurrent episodes of cystitis, which occur once or twice a month, is referred by her general practitioner. Describe your initial assessment and subsequent management.**

- *History.* This should include details regarding the frequency of infections, any precipitating or alleviating factors and the relationship to sexual intercourse. It should also be documented whether these have been proven on urine culture or if the woman has simply been treated symptomatically. Previous urinary tract infections (UTIs) as a child and a history of diabetes mellitus should also be discussed. If there is the possibility of recent foreign travel, specific questions should be asked concerning tuberculosis (TB) and schistosomiasis. Direct questions should also be asked regarding contraception and the possibility of pregnancy.                                    **(2 marks)**

- *Examination.* A complete physical examination with particular emphasis on abdominal and pelvic findings should be made. Pelvic examination should exclude the presence of a pelvic mass, urethral diverticulum, cystocele or large urinary residual.      **(2 marks)**

- *Investigations.* A urine sample should be sent for microscopy, culture and sensitivity (including fastidious organisms). Should there be a suspicion of TB or schistosomiasis, specific cultures should be sent.                                        **(2 marks)**

- A random blood sugar should be measured and, if indicated, a glucose tolerance test performed.                                                          **(2 marks)**

- A transvaginal ultrasound (TVUS) should be performed to estimate the urinary residual and exclude pelvic pathology that may impede bladder emptying, such as ovarian cysts and urethral and bladder diverticulae.                              **(2 marks)**

- Urodynamics should be performed to investigate lower urinary tract function. This will give information regarding urinary residual, flow rate and pressure–flow studies. Imaging will allow the identification of vesico-ureteric reflux, bladder and urethral diverticulae. If there is a suggestion of voiding difficulties, a urethral pressure profile should be performed to exclude a urethral stricture.                    **(2 marks)**

- Imaging of the upper urinary tract should be performed using either ultrasound or an intravenous urogram (IVU). It may be relevant here to mention the use of ultrasound as opposed to ionizing radiation.                                      **(2 marks)**

- If there is any evidence of upper tract pathology, renal function should be checked.
                                                                        **(1 mark)**

- Subsequent cystoscopy and bladder biopsy should also be undertaken to exclude any intravesical pathology such as bladder calculi, polyps or diverticulae. Cystoscopic appearances suggestive of interstitial cystitis (glommerulations, haemorrhage on refilling the bladder) should also be mentioned. Biopsy will help to differentiate between a chronic follicular cystitis affecting the mucosa and lamina propria and an interstitial cystitis affecting the deeper muscle layers.   **(2 marks)**

- *Management.* Any underlying pathology should be treated. If all investigations are unremarkable, consideration should be given to:
    review of personal hygiene
    advice regarding voiding, fluid intake and cranberry juice
    long-term low-dose prophylactic antibiotics, e.g. norfloxacin, trimethoprim or a cephalosporin
    the use of antibiotics to cover 'at-risk' activities such as intercourse
    the use of a urinary antiseptic, e.g. hexamine hippurate (Hiprex®).   **(3 marks)**
    *See Chapter 61, Lower urinary tract infections.*

**64. A 67-year-old woman presents with a history of symptomatic prolapse and occasional stress incontinence whilst coughing and sneezing. On examination by her general practitioner, she was found to have second-degree uterine descent, a moderate cystocele and mild rectocele. Describe your subsequent management.**

- A detailed history should be taken with regard to the specific symptoms of which she complains and whether they are related to the clinical findings. Concurrent medical problems and drug history should also be mentioned, as these may be responsible for exacerbation of the symptoms. Specific questions should be asked relating to her urinary symptoms and, in particular, how troublesome the symptoms of stress incontinence are. Questions regarding sexual activity, bowel symptoms (especially constipation) and the use of HRT or other drugs should also be asked.   **(2 marks)**

- Clinical assessment should include abdominal and pelvic examinations. This should involve an assessment of urogenital atrophy, examination and grading using a Simms' speculum and, if necessary, repeating the examination while standing and straining. Objective assessment using the Pelvic Organ Prolapse Quantification scoring system (POPQ) may also be performed.   **(3 marks)**

- *Investigations.* These should include midstream urine (MSU) and either simple cystometry or videocystourethrography in view of her symptoms. It is important to exclude a chronic urinary residual and detrusor over-activity and to evaluate objectively the degree of sphincter incompetence. A TVUS should also be performed to exclude intrapelvic pathology.   **(3 marks)**

- Discussion regarding the clinical and urodynamic findings and the severity of each of her symptoms should include the following.
    - The use of pelvic floor exercises with or without ring pessary as a conservative approach. This should also include alterations in lifestyle, such as avoidance of constipation, cessation of smoking and weight loss if applicable.   **(2 marks)**
    - If prolapse is the main symptom and she is not troubled by the symptoms of stress incontinence, even if urodynamics are suggestive of a minor degree of urodynamic stress incontinence, a vaginal hysterectomy and pelvic floor repair may be appropriate. However, she should be warned that this may not improve her symptom of stress incontinence and, should it get worse, she may require an additional continence procedure.   **(3 marks)**
    - If stress incontinence is troublesome and objectively demonstrated on urodynamic testing, a colposuspension may be more appropriate. Since she also complains of symptomatic prolapse, this should be combined with a total abdominal hysterectomy and bilateral salpingo-oophorectomy (she is postmenopausal). It should be mentioned that should this be the case, she may need an interval posterior repair for correction of the rectocele.   **(3 marks)**

Tension-free vaginal tape (TVT) is not suitable, as this will not deal with the symptoms of urogenital prolapse. **(1 mark)**

Anterior repair or a paravaginal repair alone is not indicated here, as there is co-existent uterine prolapse and rectocele. **(1 mark)**

Since this is primary surgery, there is no indication for the use of mesh. **(1 mark)**

- Finally, the possible complications of surgery in addition to the risk of recurrent prolapse should be discussed with the woman. **(1 mark)**

*See Chapter 62, Urogenital prolapse.*

**65. Describe the management of a 15-year-old girl attending the casualty department with lower abdominal pain and offensive vaginal discharge who is systemically unwell.**

- It is important to establish good rapport in order to gain her confidence and to obtain a reliable history. During the course of the consultation it is essential to avoid judgemental attitudes. **(1 mark)**

- The differential diagnosis, including non-gynaecological causes of lower abdominal pain in this age group, includes appendicitis, ectopic pregnancy, ovarian cyst accident, constipation, UTI, ovulation pain and endometriosis. **(4 marks)**

- The importance of an accurate history in this situation cannot be over-stressed; this includes a sexual history. Details of the latter should include whether sexual activity has begun, how many partners she has had and whether she has recently changed her partner. The presence of other symptoms and symptoms that may have been experienced by her partner may also be relevant. **(2 marks)**

- There are other important questions that should be asked. These include the date of her last menstrual period, previous history of a sexually transmitted infection (STI), dyspareunia, bowel and urinary symptoms, history of the pain itself, and the presence of vomiting and/or rigors. **(2 marks)**

- Her temperature, pulse and blood pressure should be measured and signs of other differential diagnoses looked for, although the most likely is PID, **in which case cervical excitation and peritonism might be found.** **(2 marks)**

- The first management decision to take is whether to admit for intravenous antibiotics and observation in view of her age and possible compliance issues. **(2 marks)**

- Next, it is important to consider the types of organisms necessary to cover, bearing in mind local sensitivities to *Neisseria gonorrhoeae*. **(2 marks)**

- Investigations should include a pregnancy test/hCG, blood count, erythrocyte sedimentation rate (ESR), endocervical swabs for chlamydial (cellular material) and gonococcal (cervical pus) infection. In certain situations, such as the inability to exclude an ectopic pregnancy, a laparoscopy might be considered. **(2 marks)**

- Contact tracing and partner notification/referral to genitourinary medicine is also required if an STI is confirmed. Other important issues that should be discussed include the importance of follow-up and future prevention issues: condoms and reliable hormonal contraception. **(1 mark)**

- Issues associated with an under-16-year-old girl include competence, consent, parental involvement and confidentiality. If discussing contraceptive advice, consideration should be given to the Fraser guidelines (from the Gillick case). **(2 marks)**

  *See Chapter 63.1, Infection and sexual health.*

**66. A 22-year-old woman attends your outpatient clinic, referred with an offensive vaginal discharge. She has confided to the nurse that she also has some 'lumps' on the vulva. Outline your management.**

- The problem of a young woman with a discharge and vulval swelling raises the possibility of an STI, and this should be the starting point of her management.    **(2 marks)**

- It is therefore important to adopt a non-judgemental attitude and to establish a good rapport with the patient.    **(2 marks)**

- Given the possibility of an STI, a careful sexual history is vital. This should establish whether or not she is sexually active and also details of her partner or partners.    **(2 marks)**

- Enquiry should be made about the nature of both problems, whether the discharge causes itching/irritation (e.g. in candidiasis), exacerbating factors such as sexual intercourse and bathing (e.g. in bacterial vaginosis), and cyclicity. With regard to the lesions on the vulva, it is important to ascertain how long she has had them, whether they have spread and if they are sore or are causing problems.    **(4 marks)**

- The examination should be performed considering the differential diagnosis of vulval swellings; genital warts are the most likely cause in this age group. If there is any doubt, biopsy should be performed. As sexual transmission appears likely in this case, investigations should be performed appropriately to exclude other STIs. Investigations should include endocervical and vaginal swabs for chlamydia, gonorrhoea, trichomonas and candidiasis and Amsel's criteria for bacterial vaginosis.    **(4 marks)**

- If an STI is found, such as genital warts, it is important to refer to genitourinary medicine for further investigation, treatment and contact tracing.    **(3 marks)**

- Finally, it is essential that the patient is given a clear and understandable explanation, using appropriate language, reassurances and leaflets to back up the verbal information.    **(3 marks)**

*See Chapter 63.1, Infection and sexual health.*

**67. A married couple present to the gynaecology clinic with 4 years of infertility. All preliminary investigations in primary care have been normal. During the consultation, the woman bursts into tears and admits that consummation of the marriage has never taken place. Describe what you will do next.**

- It is important not to appear shocked or angry that this has only just been disclosed. The couple should be put at ease and it should be explained to them that this is not an uncommon problem and that you will arrange some help for them but need a little more information. **(4 marks)**

- First, it is of value to understand the different causes of non-consummation. Those that should be considered in this case include male and female psychosexual problems. In the former, one might consider such problems as erectile dysfunction, premature ejaculation and decreased libido. In the female, low libido, vaginismus and problems with arousal should all be considered. Other organic causes such as vulval pain disorders and other causes of superficial dyspareunia should also be considered. **(8 marks)**

- It is essential to be able to ask some open-ended questions, such as 'What actually happens when you try to have sex?'. **(3 marks)**

- There should be a thorough exploration of each partner's background, including previous sexual history/partner, a history of assault, rape or child sex abuse. **(2 marks)**

- Once the type and context of the problem have been defined, consideration should be given to onward referral to specialized agencies. The exact type of agencies and clinicians that might be appropriate will depend upon the provisional diagnosis. **(3 marks)**

*See Chapter 63.2, Dyspareunia and other psychosexual problems.*

**68. A 14-year-old girl is referred to your clinic with heavy periods. During the consultation she appears very withdrawn and tearful. She asks to be put on 'the pill' and urges you not to tell her mother, who has temporarily left the room. What sort of issues does this presentation raise and how would you manage them?**

- Initially, there should be concern regarding her surreptitious behaviour. It is possible that she is trying to conceal something from her mother and, given her age, the possibility of child sex abuse must be considered. Alternatively, she may be in a sexual relationship that is either unknown to or forbidden by her mother. **(5 marks)**

- In such a situation, it is vital to establish good rapport with the girl. This can be achieved only through gentle handling and a gradual building of confidence. The girl should be allowed to realize that you are not forming judgements about her behaviour. **(2 marks)**

- If there is a consensual sexual relationship (unknown to the mother) with a partner of similar age, she should be informed with regard to the legal issues. These are formalized in the Fraser guidelines, which followed the Gillick case. The risks of pregnancy and STI need to be discussed with the girl, and thus the need for the use of condoms plus a reliable hormonal method of contraception. A useful consideration here would be liaison with a local young people's contraception service. Hormonal contraception may be of value in this age group in order to control menorrhagia. **(7 marks)**

- If child sex abuse is suspected (or confirmed by the girl), it is essential to involve other agencies for advice and ongoing management, but with the consent of the young woman, if possible. It is possible to obtain anonymous basic advice from the social services (child protection officer) or paediatrics in the first instance without disclosing the young woman's name. Clinical examination is not appropriate at this point, although it may be required later. **(6 marks)**

*See Chapter 63.3, Child sex abuse.*

**69. You are the on-call specialist registrar in obstetrics and gynaecology and a 32-year-old woman is referred to you by the police with a history of alleged rape and vaginal bleeding. There is no forensic medical officer available to examine this woman and you are asked to perform a forensic medical examination of the complainant and to treat her injuries. Discuss how would you manage this problem.**

- The examination should take place in an appropriate environment, with a trained female police officer present and a friend or relative of the victim, if possible.      **(1 mark)**

- The priority of the examination is to treat the victim's genital injuries or other serious injuries first.      **(1 mark)**

- Direct questions should be asked of the complainant, based upon the 'first account' obtained by the police officer, to direct forensic sampling. Relevant medical and sexual histories should be taken and the questions and answers recorded verbatim.   **(3 marks)**

- The following informed consent for the examination needs to be obtained:
    consent for a medical examination (genital and non-genital)
    consent for the collection of forensic evidence
    consent for the retention of clothing for forensic examination
    consent for disclosure of details of the medical record to the police/Crown Prosecution
        Service (CPS).      **(4 marks)**

- A 'Sexual Offences' kit should be used to perform the examination.      **(1 mark)**

- Once the genital injuries have been treated, a forensic examination should be undertaken, including:
    assessment of the emotional and physical state of the complainant
    clothes sent for forensic examination
    injuries described, documented on body charts and photographed (intimate photographs should be taken by a same-gender photographer)
    non-intimate samples – buccal swab, saliva specimen, head hair combings, skin swab, finger-nail scrapings or cuttings
    intimate samples – pubic hair combings, vulval, introital, low vaginal, cervical, high vaginal, anal, rectal swabs
    blood samples – for DNA analysis, blood typing, alcohol estimation, toxicology screen
    urine samples – for alcohol and toxicology screen
    control swabs sent with the forensic samples
    examination gown sent for forensic analysis
    the samples labelled and sent to the forensic science laboratory
    a witness statement completed.      **(7 marks)**

- Screening or treatment for sexually transmitted diseases (STDs) and postcoital contraception should be offered.                                                  **(2 marks)**

- Counselling should be offered, information provided about support agencies and follow-up arranged.                                                               **(1 mark)**

  *See Chapter 63.4, Rape and rape counselling.*

**70. A 54-year-old woman has a 3-year history of persistent pruritus vulvae that has failed to respond to repeated antifungal treatment and hydrocortisone creams. She has no history of atopy or vaginal discharge. General examination was unremarkable. On pelvic examination, the vulval skin had a parchment-like appearance, with some areas of telangiectases and loss of the normal architecture. What is the differential diagnosis? Explain which one is most likely and discuss how you would manage this problem.**

*Diagnosis*
- Given the appearances of the vulva, lichen sclerosus is the most likely diagnosis.

  **(2 marks)**

- The alternatives would include contact dermatitis, although this is unlikely as there is no history of atopy. **(1 mark)**

- Recurrent vulvovaginal candidiasis is also unlikely as there is no associated history of discharge and she is not in the usual age group for candidiasis. **(1 mark)**

- Squamous cell hyperplasia might also cause vulval pruritus. However, the findings on vulval examination do not favour a hyperplastic process, although biopsy would be necessary to fully exclude squamous cell hyperplasia. **(1 mark)**

- Finally, a diagnosis of seborrhoeic dermatitis might be considered. However, if this were the underlying problem, one would expect to see similar features on general examination, and a response to topical antifungals and weak steroids might have been anticipated. **(1 mark)**

*Management*
- The initial history and examination should include enquiry about past medical history, general health and drug exposure. General and vaginal examinations should be performed. **(2 marks)**

- With regard to specific investigation, the most important note is that biopsy is not usually required unless there are any suspicious features on the vulva. These features would include ulcerated or localized areas of hyperplasia with a raised and irregular contour. If superadded infection is present, bacteriological swabs should be taken. Glycosuria needs to be excluded. **(4 marks)**

*Explanation/information*
- It is important that the patient is given a clear explanation of the diagnosis. In particular, she should understand the chronic nature of lichen sclerosus and that the aims of treatment are primarily to control the symptoms. **(2 marks)**

- The risk of malignant progression should be raised. Currrent estimates suggest a lifetime risk of 5 per cent, but it is not possible to quantify individual risk. She should be advised to report any new symptoms or changes in vulval appearance promptly so that early biopsy can be performed as required. Information sheets should be supplied and the patient encouraged to ask questions should she not understand any of the information.

**(3 marks)**

*Treatment*

- The first-line treatment is usually with topical fluorinated corticosteroids. More than 90 per cent of patients respond to these, but most require some form of maintenance therapy with intermittent steroids and/or bland emollients. As this is a chronic condition with a potential malignancy risk, long-term follow-up either with her GP practitioner or in a hospital clinic is advisable.                                **(3 marks)**

*See Chapter 64, Benign vulval problems.*

## 71. Counsel a woman who has been given a diagnosis of vulval vestibulitis.

- Once a diagnosis of vulval vestibulitis has been made, the initial step is one of explaining it to the woman and offering reassurance that it will either resolve spontaneously (30 per cent of cases spontaneously resolve in the absence of any specific treatment) or be amenable to interventions. This is an important first step, as many sufferers are very despondent when they eventually get their diagnosis. It is important to emphasize the role that stress may play in both the genesis and continuation of symptoms. **(5 marks)**

- Initially, the woman should be advised on vulval hygiene and the use of simple, bland emollients to minimize the risk of skin drying and splitting. Aqueous cream is a suitable soap substitute in this situation. **(3 marks)**

- More specifically, it is worth prescribing local anaesthetic gels for at least a short trial. These may allow the woman to continue in a sexual relationship without feeling pain, and thereby reduce the possible risk of avoiding sex and developing sex-avoidance behaviour. **(3 marks)**

- There is little evidence that other topical applications, including steroids and other anti-inflammatory agents, are of any value. However, it is important to point out the potential risks of various creams and ointments. These can be irritant, and women should be advised to avoid such 'over-the-counter' products. **(3 marks)**

- Surgery, specifically the modified vestibulectomy, gives a 60 per cent complete response rate. Surgery should be explained in detail to the woman and it should be emphasized that it does not cause any significant cosmetic harm and can be of value in selected patients. It is essential that women understand that all other options have been tried prior to committing to surgical intervention. Following successful vestibulectomy, it is still likely that some form of sexual rehabilitation will be required, as there may be learnt reflexes and avoidance to overcome. This can be achieved through the use of dilators, psychosexual counselling and, perhaps of most importance, a supportive and well-informed partner. **(6 marks)**

*See Chapter 65, Vulval pain syndromes.*

**72.** **A 26-year-old nulliparous woman has had her second-ever cervical smear and this has been reported as moderate dyskaryosis. She is currently using combined oral contraception and is normal on examination apart from a cervical ectropion. Describe an appropriate management plan and what would be appropriate counselling for this woman.**

- She should be referred for a colposcopic examination.                                    **(3 marks)**

- If any colposcopic abnormality is seen, she should have:
    a directed biopsy or                                                                   **(2 marks)**
    excision of the transformation zone.                                                   **(1 mark)**

- If a directed biopsy confirms cervical intraepithelial neoplasia (CIN) 2 or 3, she can be treated by excision or ablation.                                                          **(3 marks)**

- If a directed biopsy confirms CIN 1 or less, surveillance is an option.                   **(3 marks)**

- At or before colposcopy, she should be reassured that cancer is unlikely.                 **(2 marks)**

- The pre-cancerous nature of the histology should be explained.                            **(2 marks)**

- The need for follow-up after treatment should be explained.                               **(2 marks)**

- There is no evidence that treatment affects fertility.                                     **(2 marks)**
  *See Chapter 66, Pre-invasive disease.*

**73. A 54-year-old woman presents with postmenopausal bleeding. She has been on tamoxifen for 2 years following treatment for a node-positive breast cancer. This tumour was oestrogen-receptor positive. Discuss counselling and her further management.**

- The reasons for prompt referral and investigation should be explained to the woman. Whilst she should be aware of the risk of endometrial pathology, she should also be reassured that no adverse pathology is found in the majority of cases.                **(2 marks)**

- The woman should be offered an explanation of the paradoxical effects of tamoxifen, in that it is anti-oestrogenic in breast tissue but has oestrogenic effects on the endometrium. Counselling should include the fact that tamoxifen use is a risk factor for endometrial adenocarcinoma and sarcoma but also for benign conditions such as endometrial hyperplasia and polyps.                **(4 marks)**

- She should continue on her tamoxifen because of the proven benefits to her survival, and changes to her treatment should be made after completion of her investigations in consultation with her breast team.                **(4 marks)**

- The investigations and their limitations are as follows.
    Transvaginal ultrasonography can be used to triage cases for further investigation but is limited by endometrial thickening and cystic atrophy, which will produce misleading appearances.                **(4 marks)**
    Outpatient endometrial sampling may be used, again as triage, as a positive result will allow treatment to be expedited . A negative biopsy will still require further investigation.                **(4 marks)**
    Hysteroscopy is the investigation of choice and targeted biopsies can be taken.                **(2 marks)**

*See Chapter 67, Endometrial cancer.*

**74. Describe the management of a 26-year-old nulliparous woman referred by a practice nurse with a cervical smear report suggesting high-grade dyskaryosis suspicious of invasive disease.**

- The woman should be referred for urgent colposcopy.                      **(1 mark)**

- The extent of any lesions should be mapped out and, if appropriate, a punch biopsy should be performed. If the lesion looks like CIN 3, an excisional procedure by large loop excision of the transformation zone (LLETZ) can be performed, removing the entire transformation zone with any endocervical extension.                      **(4 marks)**

- If the colposcopic features suggest microinvasive disease, a cold knife cone should be performed under general anaesthesia.                      **(2 marks)**

- If obvious cancer is present, a small wedge or similar-sized biopsy may suffice to confirm the diagnosis.                      **(2 marks)**

- An experienced histopathologist should evaluate the tissue. If the results demonstrate high-grade intraepithelial neoplasia only, no further treatment is necessary other than cytological follow-up.                      **(2 marks)**

- If the results demonstrate microinvasive disease down to a depth of <3 mm and horizontal spread of <7 mm with complete excision of invasive and pre-invasive disease, no further treatment is necessary other than follow-up. Lymphadenectomy is not indicated, as the risk of diseased nodes in a lesion of this size is negligible.    **(4 marks)**

- If the lesion is incompletely excised, repeat excision is warranted in case there are other invasive components present.                      **(1 mark)**

- If the lesion is >3 mm but <5 mm in depth, lymphadenectomy may be indicated, by either 'open' or laparoscopic surgery. If the lesion is completely excised, no further local treatment to the cervix is necessary.                      **(2 marks)**

- If the lesion is >7 mm in transverse diameter or 5 mm in depth of invasion, the disease is considered to be Stage Ib and radical treatment should be considered.    **(2 marks)**

*See Chapter 68, Cervical cancer.*

**75. A 25-year-old nulliparous woman presents with a tender mass arising from the pelvis and consistent in size with a 16-week gestation. Pregnancy test is negative. Ultrasound scan confirms the presence of a complex ovarian mass with features highly suspicious of malignancy. The eventual histology is that of a germ-cell tumour. Describe your management.**

- A complete history should be taken and full clinical examination performed. The supraclavicular areas need to be examined for lymphadenopathy and the chest for evidence of pleural effusions. Abdominal examination, pelvic examination and rectal examination should be performed to assess the size and mobility of the mass and to look for evidence of metastatic disease (hepatomegaly, rectal shelf). **(4 marks)**

- Investigations include measurement of alpha-fetoprotein (aFP), βhCG, CA125, urea and electrolytes, full blood count and a chest X-ray. **(2 marks)**

- Laparotomy through a mid-line incision is the treatment of choice. Free peritoneal fluid or peritoneal washings should be sent for cytology, and oophorectomy performed to remove an intact mass. The contralateral ovary should be biopsied if an abnormality is identified. A thorough assessment of all peritoneal surfaces, peritoneal biopsies, omentectomy and removal of enlarged pelvic or para-aortic nodes should be performed. **(8 marks)**

- Having diagnosed a germ-cell malignancy on histology, the patient should be referred to a medical oncologist for adjuvant combination chemotherapy (bleomycin, etoposide and cisplatin). This is not indicated in cases of dysgerminoma stage I or immature teratoma grade 1. The Macmillan nurse will be actively involved in the management and counselling of the patient. The high survival rates following treatment should be emphasized and the likelihood of future fertility discussed. **(6 marks)**

*See Chapter 69, Benign and malignant ovarian masses.*

**76. Describe the management of a 67-year-old woman presenting with a 4-week history of a painful 3.5 cm vulval ulcer close to the clitoris.**

- A full clinical examination should be performed to assess the involvement of surrounding structures such as the urethra and vagina. The groins and supraclavicular area should be examined for lymphadenopathy.                                         **(4 marks)**

- The cervix should be examined to exclude a co-existing cervical cancer. Investigations should include a full blood count and urea and electrolytes. A pelvic ultrasound should be arranged to exclude any other gynaecological pathology.                        **(4 marks)**

- The lesion should be biopsied, including the edge of the tumour and the deep tissue to assess the depth of invasion. Excision biopsy should be avoided, as this could interfere with subsequent management planning.                                          **(4 marks)**

- Surgery will be the treatment of choice, with at least a wide radical local excision of the cancer aiming to remove a 1 cm disease-free margin. Bilateral inguinal node dissection through separate incisions should be performed to include the nodes below the cribriform fascia and medial to the femoral vein.                                      **(6 marks)**

- Adjuvant radiotherapy should be considered if two or more inguinal nodes are involved with cancer or there is evidence of extracapsular spread.                               **(2 marks)**

  *See Chapter 70, Vulval and vaginal cancer.*

## 77. Describe the acute gynaecological management of suspected molar pregnancy.

- Most molar pregnancies present with a history similar to that of threatened or incomplete miscarriage (vaginal blood loss after a period of amenorrhoea). Initial investigations, after establishing haemodynamic stability, should include pelvic ultrasound scanning, which will yield a characteristic snowstorm appearance. If the diagnosis of a molar pregnancy is suspected, a quantitative βhCG should be taken, as this will aid monitoring of disease progression.                                    **(6 marks)**

- Many complete moles will be diagnosed by this means. Suction curettage is the treatment of choice, all evacuated tissue being sent for histopathological examination. The use of oxytocic drugs is best avoided unless life-threatening bleeding occurs. In the case of partial mole, the diagnosis is often not made until the histopathology of evacuated uterine contents is reported. In 90 per cent of all cases of molar pregnancy, suction curettage is all that is needed as treatment.                              **(6 marks)**

- In the remaining 10 per cent, gestational trophoblastic disease persists and may require further intervention. This is the main reason why the RCOG has established a national registration and monitoring system for all presumed cases of molar pregnancy. With persistent gestational trophoblastic disease, there may be a role for second evacuation after discussion with the screening centre; often, however, particularly where hCG levels are high and there is evidence on ultrasound scan of invasive mole, these patients need to be transferred to the specialist centre for potentially curative chemotherapy.

    **(5 marks)**

- Hysterectomy is only occasionally performed in the acute management of molar pregnancy – rarely, this may be unavoidable for acute complications (unstoppable haemorrhage or major perforation) or on the wishes of the older patient who has completed her family.                                                            **(3 marks)**

*See Chapter 71, Gestational trophoblastic disease.*

# Index